trotman

Music Industry

UNCOVERED

2ND EDITION

To Steve

Music Industry Uncovered
This second edition published in 2007 by Trotman
an imprint of Crimson Publishing
Westminster House, Kew Road, Richmond TW9 2ND
www.crimsonpublishing.co.uk

First edition published 2004 by Trotman and Co Ltd
Reprinted 2006

Author Tania Shillam

Designed by XAB

British Library Cataloguing in Publication Data
A catalogue record for this book is available from the British
Library

ISBN 978 1 84455 132 3

Typeset by Mac Style, Nafferton, East Yorkshire
Printed and bound in Great Britain by
Creative Print & Design, Wales

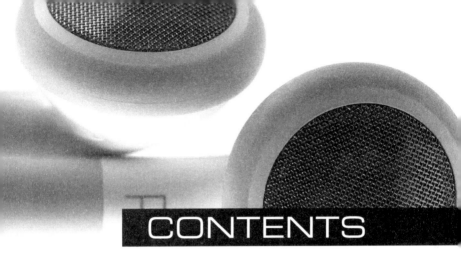

CONTENTS

About the author

My involvement in music reached a peak as a presenter of an arts and culture radio show. In between the interviews, I played as much old soul, funk, disco and blues as I could fit in. I have rediscovered magical orchestrations of seemingly innocent pop songs and found unusual back stories to musicians I thought I knew.

I have had long, indulgent interviews with many artists including Jazzman Terrance Blanchard who scores the music for Spike Lee's films, soul voice extraordinaire Natalie Williams, Andrew Love Levy from The Brand New Heavies and Katie Melua in her dressing room before her Wembley Stadium concert. On the red carpet at the Brit Awards, when iconic stars of the moment make their way into the evening of celebration, I've interviewed Jazzy B, Girls Aloud, McFly, Dave from The Killers, Amy Winehouse, Natasha Beddingfield, Will Young ... and many more.

I was presenting in the Christmas week of James Brown's untimely death and therefore played track after track after funky track from the Godfather of Soul. I asked almost every interviewee in subsequent weeks what they remembered of the moment they heard the news.

I've immersed myself in the best music as a result of being a radio presenter. I've discovered new bands, rediscovered favourites and oozed about my feelings for music on air to my listeners. Emails reached the show requesting tracks from old Funk bands I'd never heard of and so I continue to be a grateful student.

I love writing career guidance books. I've watched people's eyes sparkle as they remember their attempts to break into their area of the music industry and I try to convey that excitement to the reader through my writing. They all believe very deeply in passing on advice and helping teenagers to find their footing and their confidence. I hope I've done their words justice.

Acknowledgements

I'm very privileged and grateful for the help of Publishing Director Mina Patria; also to Seltzer Cole for his daily and indefatigable interest and support; and to all those who feature in this book:

- Moshik from the band Moshikop

- The Dualers

- Neil Ward-Dutton from the band Clear

- Andrea Terrano, founder, manager and owner of Iguana Studios

- Neil Gardener, Gateway School of Recording and Music Technology

- Music producer Ahmad Dayes

- Music producer Tai Newsam (aka Shredda)

- Alice Schofield of Anglo Plugging

- Ludes' band manager Sam Eldridge

- Oliver X, formerly of EMI

- Dave VJ from Choice FM

- Laure Panerai, music director for Momo's

- Larmer Tree Festival co-director Julia Safe

- James Feniman, manager of Four Kornerz

- Daryl Easlea of Universal Music and author of *Everybody Dance: Chic and the Politics of Disco*

Thank you to Propellerhead Software for permission to reprint a screenshot of Reason. Please note that Reason, ReCycle, ReBirth, ReFills, ReWire, and REX are either registered trademarks or trademarks of Propellerhead Software in the UK and/or other countries.

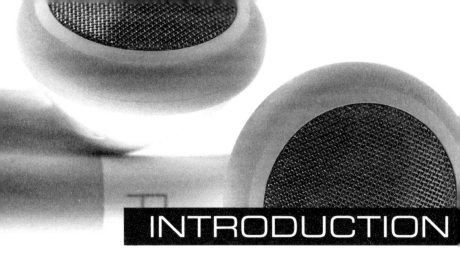

INTRODUCTION

The music industry makes money by the truckload! It's a place where very sharp, talented people congregate. It is also a monster of greed and the pitfalls are plentiful. If you want to join this industry then you need to keep up to date with the changes that are taking place as well as following and predicting trends to figure out how the industry can adapt to them.

WHY READ THIS BOOK?

If you are looking for a career in mainstream music, this book offers you a better understanding of:

● the role you are going for

● where to get information and what kinds of questions to ask

● the access points to your chosen career

● the various jobs in the music industry and how they interact.

In this book you will find interviews with professionals who will help you on your way. The advice given is their advice. They will show you the steps to take and give examples of work. Their experiences will highlight both the good and the bad.

The examples, tips and anecdotes written on these pages will give you a clear idea of the various careers and how to get one, as well as a few signposts to point you in the direction of other possibilities. To demystify the industry, you will find illustrations of:

- the traditional record company structure

- the old and new music-making process and the jobs involved

- where to find traditional work experience placements

- established job profiles to give you a taster of the variety of jobs

- the 'brave new world' of technology and new opportunities.

Plenty of people are leaving the business because traditional roles are being squeezed out, but plenty of people are entering the industry through modern technology. Affordable music-making technology and the internet have really rocked the boat, which means that new roles are materialising.

You are looking for a career in a very competitive industry but there are many people who have found spectacular success while still in their teens.

- Katie Melua sold more than 350,000 albums and had a five-album deal worth £2 million by the time she was 19 years old.

- Amy Winehouse founded her first rap group when she was around 10 years old. At 12 years old she attended the Sylvia Young Theatre School but was expelled a year later for 'not applying herself'. She later attended the Brit School and received her first guitar at 13 years old. By the time she was 16 years old, she was discovered and began singing professionally. In 2007 she made chart history as the highest debuting British female artist ever in the US album chart with the album *Back to Black*.

- Lily Allen, born in Hammersmith, west London, in 1985, found her fame through the use of MySpace. In 2002, her demo caught the attention of Warner Music and Allen was signed to a deal, but it turned out to be a fruitless one. Three years later, the artist signed with Regal Records. When she and the label couldn't agree on a sound for her, Allen started posting her demos on her MySpace page, where she also wrote candid updates about developments in her life and career.

● Joss Stone was 14 years old when she tried out for the British television talent show *Star for a Night*. Auditioning for record labels in New York came next and by the time she was 16 years old, she was a teenage soul diva. She was a girl from Devon yet sang like 'the second coming of Gladys Knight'. It caused a lot of debate. She is quoted as saying that one label executive remarked that he 'would never sign a white girl with a black girl's voice'. In 2007 her album *Introducing Joss Stone* debuted at number two on the Billboard album chart with sales of 118,000. It was the highest new entry by a British female artist in US album chart history.

● Tai Newsam (aka Shredda) of Teenage Testimony has written of his experiences as a producer in Chapter 4 of this book (see pages 46–50). He started as a 14-year-old schoolboy with the support of a teacher. After two years of dedicated self-teaching he is producing rap, hip hop and garage, and has the ambition to create a new genre of music and to have his own record label.

However, fame and success are elusive to the majority of people entering the industry so they plod through the years into their twenties and thirties. With music as a passion, 'Plan B' is a must to guard against the inevitable knocks.

But if you have ambition, talent and tenacity you will make it!

FASCINATING FACT

In the UK alone, the music industry employs over 130,000 people in various sectors including numerous technology start-ups, investors, artists, record companies, media operators, content service providers, site owners, and marketing and advertising companies. The industry contributes £5 billion to the economy.
***Source:* Bipin Parmar, www.thechilli.com**

WHY YOU?

Do you have an enviable collection of vinyl and CDs? Are you a 'download demon'? Do you devour the music magazines and follow bands or individuals through their concerts and trials and tribulations? If so, you'll know at first hand how successful the industry is in contributing to the flavour of our lives. It is really incredibly powerful.

Plotting your way into your career starts here. Be clear about the talents that you have to offer and what your achievements have been so far. More people want to be part of the scene than the scene will accommodate so you have to put yourself ahead.

The successful people live and breathe the industry. They all obsess about music, fashions, trends and images. People really do live for their music.

The question is: Do you? What is your involvement in music now? Are you producing tracks in your spare time? Do you seek out unsigned bands at college or in pubs and clubs or on the internet? Do you write about new trends for your school newspaper? Who inspires you?

TASK: PLANNING YOUR CAREER

Write a paragraph about why you would like to pursue this career. Refine it as you work your way through this book. This is pretty difficult to get right but put down the first description that comes to your pen. Project into the near future, if you like, of what you would *like* to write; in other words, what you would like to have achieved in a year or two.

The following are example paragraphs.

● I have been producing tracks for download for two years and advertise my skills via MySpace, Flickr, Bebo and Facebook. I specialise in rap, hip hop and garage. I have created my own website which is a platform to sell my work. My ambition is to work with artists such as Lilly Allen and Amy Winehouse.

- I have been lead singer with my band for a year, having met through the local borough orchestra. We have played concerts at the local Party in the Park and at the borough's Guy Fawkes celebrations and regularly play at a neighbourhood venue which specialises in soul and blues music.

- I have been promoting bands for three years and have set up a client list of unsigned artists to showcase in local venues. I have a college place to do a diploma in advertising and marketing to begin in the next semester. In the meantime I am organising my first foreign tour to Germany to promote three nights in Berlin. I am a member of the Music Managers' Forum.

Whatever it is that you've been doing in pursuit of your career, write it down as if you are introducing yourself. At some point a potential employer will ask you to justify your application. Anticipate all the questions an employer might have and rehearse the answers. A good way of preparing for an interview is to write down interview questions and think through the strongest way to put your answers, including exciting examples.

Examples are important. If you say that you *think* you might be good at 'such-and-such' and that you *think* you might like to do 'so-and-so', faces will fall, big sighs will be heard and you'll be shown the door. Have proof that you know what you are talking about.

If you haven't made a start on your music career yet, don't be daunted. Make a start now. Create a page on a social networking site and start a blog. Write a review of the latest CD you bought/downloaded and, hey presto, you're a music journalist in the making!

CAREER RESEARCH

If you don't already have a clear idea of where your career will be, ask yourself a few more questions. Do you picture yourself in a studio, office or venue? Do you think of live music, television entertainment or internet streaming? Where do you get your music from: on the high street or online? Are you laptop active? What images do you conjure up when you think of the British music industry? You could start to do the following research:

- if you see yourself becoming an industry executive, then read everything you can about the major companies and small labels and how they are evolving

- if you see yourself as a producer, find out about the access points to the industry and the route other producers have taken

- if you want to be a band member, find out what skills you need to make yourself indispensable.

As you work your way through this book, think about where your passion lies and where you belong. Keep an open mind about jobs in the industry that might help you towards the desired end result. If you are offered work experience by your school at the opposite end of the industry to the place you want to end up, it can be a good thing. Be flexible and think laterally.

A broad understanding of the industry will help you to work out a career strategy. The profile of Oliver X (see pages 62–65) shows how many years he spent outside the industry gathering crucial skills, all of which finally led to his dream job.

SOURCES OF CAREER INFORMATION

When you approach people for advice, from the school careers officer to the teacher to the industry contact, be clear about what help you want. In other words, make it easy for people to help you.

Make yourself familiar with general sources of career information. Here are a couple of examples:

- the BBC 'One Life' website (www.bbc.co.uk/onelife) gives career and work placement advice; also covers applications, CVs and interviews

- the BBC Radio 1 'One Music' website (www.bbc.co.uk/radio1/ onemusic) gives profiles of jobs such as: artist and repertoire (A&R) scouts; artist manager; tour manager; journalist; studio engineer; and PR (public relations)/promotion manager

- the British Recorded Music Industry's *Music Education Directory* offers 'those considering a career in the music industry a single point of reference for all relevant education'; the website (www.bpi-med.co.uk) provides a series of maps of the four key sectors of the music industry (the record company, publishing company, artist management and live-performance sectors)

● illustrations of Warner Music's company structure and career opportunities can be found on their website (www.warnermusiccareers.com).

More career sources can be found in Chapter 9.

CAREER STRATEGY

Think about what you like, what you are good at and what interests you. What do you want most from work? Pick your top priorities from the list below:

● to be **creative**: you could be an artist, a producer, an illustrator or perhaps a website founder

● to earn big **money**: the highest earning executives are to be found at the helm of the major labels

● to be an inspiring **boss**: this is also a personality trait that suits teaching and mentoring

● to be **independent**: as a freelance worker you have to manage your finances and tax returns as well as your career

● to be **acknowledged**: join a band (there's nothing like the applause of fans!)

● to **travel**: go on the road with a band or pursue a career in international marketing

● to develop a **portfolio career***: for the multi-skilled entrepreneur

● to have a **structured day**: a successful business has many coveted nine-to-five jobs, from accountant to personal assistant

● to have an **unstructured work life**: journalists often boast that no two days are the same

- to be **inspired**: a good radio producer finds ideas everywhere; a good press officer will find hundreds of ways to market a product; brilliant technical/computer whizz-kids are driving the industry

- to be a **troubleshooter**: you could be a consultant

- to **achieve** something every day: studio managers and producers help bands achieve the best possible sound.

---

* A portfolio career is one where, rather than working for one company, you take on various projects and cultivate several clients.

CONCLUSION

There is a huge difference between falling helplessly into mediocre job after mediocre job and putting some thought into your moves and their outcomes to ultimately achieve your fulfilment. Make a game plan.

Try writing the CV that you want to be true in ten years' time. Determine your best skills, medium talents and smallest abilities, and chart your goal.

> ### FASCINATING FACTS
>
> **TRIVIA**
> **The longest note held by a singer: this record is held by Morten Harket, lead singer with pop group a-ha. In 'Summer Moved On' (which reached No 33 in June 2000), he holds a vocal note for 20.2 seconds.**
>
> **The runner-up, and the man responsible for the longest note held on a solo single, is Bill Withers. In his 1978 hit 'Lovely Day', he holds a vocal note for 18 seconds.**
>
> **The longest title of a hit (in UK charts): this record is held by The Faces (Rod Stewart) with the hit 'You Can Make Me Dance, Sing Or Anything (Even Take the Dog for a Walk, Mend a Fuse, Fold Away the Ironing Board, or Any Other Domestic**

Shortcomings)' which has 115 letters (punctuation doesn't count!). It reached No 12 in 1974.

Record for palindromes: 'SOS' by Abba is the only palindromic hit song by a palindromic artist.

The Cross Cultural Craziness record: held by the German pop/dance trio Sash!, they are the only act to have hits in four different languages. In 1997/8 they made the Top 40 with 'Encore Une Fois' (in French), 'Ecuador' (in Spanish), 'Stay' (in English) and 'La Primavera' (in Italian). Sash!'s 1999 hit 'Colour The World' was sung in English, but it contained African lyrics by Nigerian vocalist Dr Alban and also featured Finnish singer Inka.

Source: www.everyhit.com

CHAPTER 1

Preparation

KEEP INFORMED: MUSIC AND MAINSTREAM PRESS

The music press can influence what happens in the industry and can keep tabs on the cultural changes taking place. Artists hope to promote themselves through these publications because of their substantial voice.

The major magazines of the industry have their own awards events, they sponsor gigs and festivals. Many have a dynamic online presence and some have such brand recognition that they have expanded their marketing possibilities to ownership of a radio station and/or television channel.

While some magazines are expanding into every possible media outlet, others struggle to grow. *Smash Hits* was a major name in the 1980s but recently stopped producing its printed form altogether and went over entirely to its website edition.

If music journalism is your target career you should gain as much knowledge as you can about online publications and what production skills will be needed. Look at page layouts and design, as well as website layouts and style, and find out what design and production programs are most commonly used.

INDUSTRY PRESS

The following is a taster of the major music magazines, journals and websites.

- *Kerrang!* (www.kerrang.com): born in 1981, *Kerrang!* calls itself 'the world's biggest selling weekly rock magazine', also stating: '*Kerrang!* is a television station, an awards ceremony, the co-promoter of the annual K-Fest gigs, and now a website'.

- *Mojo* (www.mojo4music.com): targeting a male audience and the older 'more discerning' reader of 25 to 45 years old, *Mojo* is an 'authoritative resource' and entertaining all-round music magazine with a great website.

- *Music Tank* (www.musictank.co.uk): calls itself 'the UK's music business network', and aims 'to give artists, managers, labels, publishers, promoters, audio professionals, press and beyond the connectivity to share ideas, exchange information and forge new partnerships – whatever the genre'. The website features all kinds of information, including the pages 'Industry Facts and Figures' and 'Training and Education'.

- *New Musical Express (NME)* (www.nme.com): a premier British music weekly which targets 15- to 35-year-olds, with two-thirds of its audience being male. *NME* has a very proud history and has been the training ground of many famous journalists, especially those from the punk era such as Tony Parsons and Julie Burchill, as well as DJ Steve Lamacq and radio presenter Danny Baker. Since the beginnings of rock 'n' roll and every emergent trend since, it has served its readership with the writings of journalists who have been proud of their craft and very passionate about their music.

- *Q* (www.q4music.com): launched in October 1986, *Q* calls itself 'the UK's best-selling serious music publication and the first choice for big-name interviews'. As well as music news and reviews, the website claims that its goal has always been to 'raise the game of music journalism'.

- *Uncut* (www.uncut.net): the publisher (IPC Media) says about the magazine: 'A must for the serious music fan, *Uncut* looks at both classic artists that have stood the test of time along with new musicians and underground trends worth notice. [The] magazine features consistently strong writing, hundreds of music and movie reviews, interviews, news, and a complimentary compilation CD with each issue.'

Find out which magazines have the largest circulations and ask yourself who they are targeting. This is an indication of where the advertisers are happy to invest their money and promote their goods. It is an indication of who has the money to buy the CDs and the expensive concert tickets. You need to consider the market carefully.

- Is it the male mid-aged market?

- Is it the teen market?

- Is it in the pages of the ethnic press?

- Is it the celebrity gossip-loaded titles?

TASK: DEVELOP AN INDUSTRY OVERVIEW

Create a cuttings scrapbook or folder to keep those press articles that have interested you the most. If you see or hear an interview on television or radio that catches your imagination then enter the name of the person and what they said in your scrapbook.

You may well get to meet that person before long, so be prepared to make good use of their company by being well informed. Develop your opinions about the characters in the industry and the changes taking place.

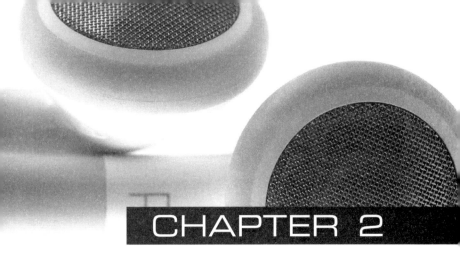

CHAPTER 2

Structure of the industry

DEPARTMENT CONNECTIONS

An excellent place to inform yourself about the structure of the music industry is the website of the BPI (British Recorded Music Industry, www.bpi.co.uk). The website www.bpi-med.co.uk has five extremely helpful maps and flow charts of key areas of the industry. Learning how one job feeds into another is the key to finding out about how the industry works. The figure below shows the different processes involved in introducing an artist (and their product) to the general public.

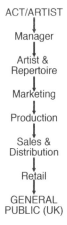

ACT/ARTIST

↓

Manager

↓

Artist & Repertoire

↓

Marketing

↓

Production

↓

Sales & Distribution

↓

Retail

↓

GENERAL PUBLIC (UK)

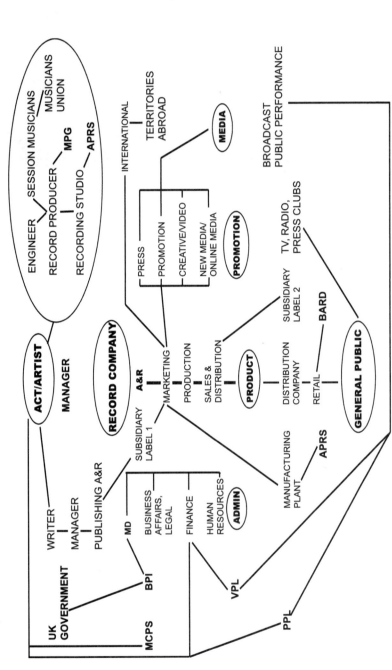

A&R: artist and repertoire; APRS: Association of Professional Recording Services; BARD: British Association of Record Dealers; BPI: British Phonographic Industry; MCPS: Mechanical Copyright Protection Society; MD: managing director; MPG: Music Producers Guild (UK); PPL: Phonographic Performances Limited; VPL: Video Performances Limited

'The British Recorded Music Industry is the British record industry's trade association. Its membership comprises of hundreds of music companies including all four "major" record companies, associate members such as manufacturers and distributors, and hundreds of independent music companies representing literally thousands of labels.'

British Recorded Music Industry (BPI)

The map of a typical UK record company (see previous page) is a close illustration of what you will find on the BPI site. You can see how all your responsibilities will relate to colleagues and adjacent departments. Knowing how various jobs and careers fit together gives you a greater understanding of a record company.

Other maps on the BPI site are: UK publishing company, artist management, live performance and music industry statistics.

JOB TITLES

Some of the most popular jobs in the music industry are:

- **the artist**: being a DJ, solo act, producer or part of a band: it depends on your skill

- **artist and repertoire (A&R)**: finding and nurturing new talent

- **artist manager**: negotiating contracts and guiding artists' careers

- **business affairs**: negotiating contracts and dealing with legal and accounting issues

- **concert promoter**: managing performances and booking the bands and the venues

- **music agent**: managing national and international performances

- **music journalist**: writing, reporting and broadcasting

- **new media**: running a website

- **plugging**: promoting the new releases to DJs and music television

- **press officer**: organising promotions and answering enquiries from the media

- **production**: packaging the product and delivering it to the retailer

- **publishing**: collecting copyright fees and royalties for the songs

- **studio manager**: organising recording sessions.

The Warner Music careers website (www.warnermusiccareers.com) has the following illustration of the music business for their graduate scheme. It gives an indication of the areas of their business to which the graduates will be 'exposed'. When you click on one of the departments a description of the work pops up and it also describes the kind of skills you need to work there.

	Artist & Repertoire	
Finance & Royalties		Business Affairs
Stategic Marketing	Human Resources Facilites Information Technology Artist Relations	Marketing
International		Press & Promotion
	Commercial	

Of course, going to university and getting onto a graduate scheme may not be for you, especially if you've been busy producing or playing in a band or being a DJ. The people interviewed in this book are from a mixture of backgrounds: some have degrees and others went straight into their careers.

RELATED ROLES
There is such a wide range of behind-the-scenes roles. Take a look at the industry magazines and periodicals. All of them have jobs pages and you can keep yourself up to date by looking at what jobs are available and how you can get a job in one area and then progress to another.

The industry survives on legions of secretaries and accountants. If you enter a record company at that level you will have transferable skills to take you to the area you want to target.

Sony BMG has a job vacancy list that you can download from their website (www.sonybmgmusic.co.uk). A typical list will include:

- analyst, financial planning and analysis: RCA Label Group

- assistant

- designer/programmer

- digital marketing assistant

- information technology support analyst

- personal assistant (PA)

- PA/accounts payable assistant

- trainee finance analyst.

You can then send your CV to be added to their recruitment database, which is used as the basis for all their external recruitment needs.

Their job page is also well worth reading for its general advice, and for their profile of an ideal candidate. The guidance offered there echoes the sentiments in this book.

There is a huge range of jobs to be had in the industry, not, of course, forgetting about the frontline artist. This is what the industry hinges on. The next chapter gives profiles of bands and the work that goes on behind the scenes to make the product.

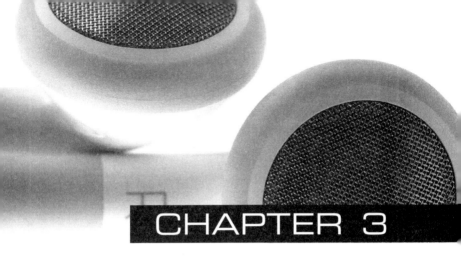

CHAPTER 3

The band, the CDs and the money

LIVE THE DREAM

Here is a taste of what driving motivation and boundless energy people apply to their music making. Bands that have the backing of the music industry fill our newspapers, magazines and television or radio programmes every day. We would be in short supply of megastars if not for the mighty record companies. However, many stars of tomorrow are finding ways to make their living and live their dream without industry backing.

The first profile is about the band Moshikop. It shows the concerns of a new band with a unique direction. The industry seems to have an endless appetite for boy bands and girl bands but many artists will resist such pressures.

'The most important thing I learn is: I always have more to learn.'

Moshik of Moshikop

The second profile is about a band called The Dualers who play on the streets of London, selling CDs direct to their audience. The final profile is from Neil Ward-Dutton of the band Clear, whose fans helped to finance their CD: his advice is about recording, pressing and distributing CDs without the backing of a label.

This chapter is full of numbers (*thousands* of CDs; *millions* of fans), so while we are swimming in figures the chapter ends with a definition of single and album sales, from Silver to Double Platinum.

MOSHIK OF MOSHIKOP

The audience were rapt at the first ever concert of Moshikop: the band was newly formed and so their experiences were new. Moshikop (www.myspace.com/moshikop) took its name from the lead member, Moshik, who is also the writer/producer. On stage he plays drums and percussion. He has already brought out a CD with Forte Records (a techno/electro label) in Germany and, as a way of making money, is a sound engineer for another band, Oi Va Voi, which had KT Tunstall as guest vocalist on their first album (www.oi-va-voi.com).

Music journalists always ask bands how they met and formed. This is a question that allows the journalist and the reader to compare the band with great bands of the past and to put them into context. We learn about their experience or naiveté; whether they picked up guitars and copied chords from Beatles records, graduated from music college or dropped out of art college.

How did you form a band?

'I was doing my first gigs by myself, which I found boring and uninspiring so I started looking for a way to make it more live even though my music is very computer based. Some of the band's members are professional musicians who play with others, some are good friends. The band I want to create should be based on unconditional granting with no ego involved; therefore I would rather be surrounded by people I love than session musicians.'

What training do you have?

'I always had a strong passion for music. As a child I felt school was a waste of time. I quit high school at 15 years old without having a specific direction; just the idea of making music. I started working in a PA company as a roadie, bought my first drum kit and I joined bands and singers to play, produce, compose, record and mix their albums and live shows. I don't have any formal qualification; I picked up drumming, producing, programming and sound engineering over the years, so you can say I'm self-taught.'

[A self-taught person is exceptionally driven and often has money to invest in the kind of equipment needed as basic tools of the trade. Moshik doesn't seem to be the kind of person who needs the help and encouragement of a teacher and a structured course. Be careful, though, if you think that dropping out of school is a good idea. Even people with extraordinary talents, the best contacts in the industry, an upbringing crammed with music appreciation courtesy of their parents, and parental money don't drop out of school. These blessed people also end up looking for volunteering work and getting breaks by showing their knowledge and enthusiasm. Diligence at school or college is a good training for industriousness in the workplace.]

Where is your base? Where do you record?
'I've got my own home studio, which allows me to work whenever I want. I can wake up in the middle of the night with an idea and put it down straight away. I record only when I feel inspired but at the same time I need to have discipline.'

What are the advantages and disadvantages of being your own boss?
'Being your own boss is the biggest freedom and at the same time it doesn't allow you to fit yourself into any routine. Working in the music industry is one of the most unstable jobs a person can get. I can find myself touring with one band, rehearsing and performing with another, producing a remix, and composing a score for a play all in one month, having no time to spend with my girlfriend, and a month later having more free time than actual work. But I love doing many different things. It keeps me alert and up to date on what's going on in different scenes.'

How do you define your music and what is your target audience?

'I don't have a target and don't like to think "yeah, I should put down a hip hop track now". I started writing my music as a therapy. This is my only place to express unreachable feelings. I don't really try to define my music as it's just too eclectic. I love to call it electro-blues, even though it's not a formal definition. I believe it's more of a crossover of down-tempo electronic and acoustic beats with some Mediterranean flavours. I can't put my finger on any particular influence. I listen to loads of genres. It's not about what music I listen to, it's about what it makes me feel.'

You are also a sound engineer for Oi Va Voi: what do you learn from going on tour with another band?

'Oi Va Voi are great musicians and above all amazing people. The most important thing I learn is: I always have more to learn; keeping my mind open to new ideas, and new or old music. That's what I love; it's all part of the big game, getting to know new people and how to get along with them, wherever they're coming from.'

You have already brought out a CD in Germany, and it didn't suit your taste. How would you do it differently?

'Today I'm looking for a label that's dedicated to something more similar to what I do; something I can feel more attached to than Forte Records. I worked on my second album for two years on and off. Finding a label would have pushed me to shape my final touch to it.'

Who else do you need in your entourage? A manager? An agent?

'I don't have a manager but I know I need one. My music is not mainstream or radio friendly so it'll be much harder for me to find one who knows how to deal with my stuff. There is an agent who helps me to find gigs, but, again, I'm not falling into a category like "world music" or "electronic" which makes it difficult to place it in these sorts of festivals or events.'

What difference has new technology and the internet made to your experience of the music industry?
'New technology gave me, as an individual, the opportunity to create most of my music by myself, using virtual instruments alongside acoustic instruments, allowing me to manipulate sounds and having unlimited tools I could otherwise never afford. On the other hand you see more people ripping off music from the internet. It's damaging us, the musicians, directly, but I see no point fighting it. It's the beginning of an individualistic and free music-making trade market. It is still early days though; it will take more than a decade for us to see where it goes.'

From Moshik's experiences, we can conclude that:

- signing to a label might help with the creative process for an artist

- a manager with empathy for the artist's genre might be hard to come by

- the nature of some music may make it challenging for an agent to place an artist in venues and festivals.

Therefore, if you are planning to be the agent or manager of a new band, you should consider the following questions.

- Will this band appeal to the kind of audience for which your record company caters?

- Are you reminded of another artist of this type who has proven that there is a large following ready to be tapped?

- Where are the venues, festivals, radio stations and DJs that will follow your instinct?

SI AND TYBER CRANSTOUN OF THE DUALERS

Brothers Si and Tyber Cranstoun are a busking duo from Croydon in south London, where they play ska music on the streets. Their father was a promoter of ska back in the 1960s (Bill Cranstoun's Savoy Sound System). Upon leaving school the brothers pursued music as a career in different ways. Si became a busker, whereas Tyber attended the Guildhall School of Music and Drama. After some television success, Tyber joined his brother singing on the streets, playing straight to the audience. The audience buy CDs direct from the artist, and this is how they got into the UK charts. The brothers also perform at their own concerts in clubs and theatres.

An article about The Dualers (on www.2-4-7-music.com) quotes them as saying: 'The only thing they didn't tell you was that music was more than just writing songs and getting on stage: it was about being there on time; releasing something on time; being famous on time'.

The Dualers have no record contract, agent or manager, and no one to distribute their material. They sell their CDs at their gigs and on the streets and in 2003 their debut single 'Kiss on the Lips' entered the charts at No 21. Then the industry showed an interest. The brothers appeared on television for *Children In Need*. A record company wanted to sign them and turn them into Robson & Jerome. This is a good example of how the lure of the coveted contract and promise of fame might not be appropriate.

The brothers are very proud of their go-it-alone approach and of the fact that they have an authentic fan base with which they have actual contact.

'In terms of how we cultivated ourselves as artists, we were, and still are, buskers, and we got our audience by collecting peoples' emails over five or six years. So it's quite a unique situation; actual people, and actual sales, so we're more the traditional "If you like us, then buy our single" band.'

Their advice is: 'If you basically have a good song, and you enjoy playing and performing, then you'll cut it. Music should always be about the music'.

'The Dualers perform a unique blend of ska, soul and reggae that appeals to all ages. They have a fan base approaching 10,000 members but have probably been seen by in excess of 4 million people while busking around south-east England for the last eight years. They have sold over 35,000 copies of their first two CDs on the streets alone.'

www.thedualers.com

The final profile is of Neil Ward-Dutton, the driving force and lead singer in a band called Clear. Moshik was thinking about the uses of a manager, an agent and the creative possibilities of being with a label; The Dualers brothers Tyber and Si are confident that self-management is better than industry interference; Neil's concerns are in another direction: which studio, which lawyer, whose money?

NEIL WARD-DUTTON OF CLEAR
Clear have a substantial fan base, which has enabled them to cut and finance their own CD. The venture was featured on BBC 2's *Working Lunch*.

Did you decide to cut a CD when you had tested the material at gigs or did you write especially for the CD?
'We'd played around half of the songs for a year or so at gigs. Overall, we rehearsed around 20 songs in total. This was mainly for time reasons, because we all hold down day jobs as well as being in a band.

'We'd been together for six years or so before we did the album, so we'd done an awful lot of gigs by the point we started. I think we probably wrote, played and then ditched well over 30 songs before we even got to the point of considering songs for recording.'

How big a part did audience feedback play?

'We relied a fair bit on audience feedback. Most bands that survive longer than a couple of years end up with some pretty loyal fans. But you've got to be careful, and make sure you don't take too much notice of your most ardent fans. Why? Because they'll love what you do, even if it's not very good. It's actually very important to get the views of someone who's at least partly independent, but who's got experience.'

Do you have a manager or agent to help with decisions?

'This is where most would turn to a manager or agent for help. We didn't have one, but we did have the help of an experienced producer/musician, Andy Metcalfe [who is perhaps best-known as a member of Squeeze in the 1980s].'

How was the fan-financing achieved?

'It happened by accident. A fan asked if the band were planning to produce a CD and offered to "lend" a couple of hundred pounds. The band members happened to mention the conversation to someone else ... who also offered to lend money. The whole thing snowballed. In the end about 40 people offered money. Clear then set up a company and made the "fans" investors. That's how the money was raised and the fans stood to share any profits.'

How many CDs did you cut?

'We manufactured 1000 copies initially. Most manufacturers will do runs of fewer than 1000 (say 500), but when you're paying for 500 you might as well go for 1000 – the unit price drops considerably as you get to 1000 units.'

Is it difficult to find a distributor?

'This is a very specialised area and it is difficult to get a distributor to be interested in you. We took the album to a few labels and one, Invisible Hands Music (ihm), was interested in helping to distribute. They already had a relationship with a distributor so the matter was made relatively easy for us.

'Distributors like predictability. Think about the job they have to do: they are gambling that they can get the right number of records to the right number of outlets at the right time. They study the CD's airplay and marketing, work out which retailers have an interested market and predict the probable stock required by the various retailers.

'They also operate on a sale or return basis. The distributor makes sure the retailer gets exactly what they need at the right time. If they get this wrong, they get the CDs back to clog up their warehouses.'

When does a band sort out the legalities?
'We've never hired a lawyer ourselves. ihm has the services of a commercial consultant (the ex-managing director of Factory Records) who helped us put together a very simple contract.'

You're not the first to be less than keen on taking the legal route. Why is this? Is it awkward to draw up a contract between friends?
'We considered it, in case of questions about royalties. We ended up drawing up a contract between ourselves in which we agreed to split everything equally, regardless of who wrote and who sang and who played.

'It's important that everyone is clear about what the position is. For example, what if one of the band members begins to write for someone else? Registering with MCPS [Mechanical Copyright Protection Society] or PRS [Performing Rights Society] means that you've taken a step into the administrative details but it's only when things go wrong that you need a lawyer.

'If you're going to go for a signing with a record company then you'll need to engage a lawyer to go through your contracts.

You don't need to engage a lawyer on a retainer. [A retainer means that you pay them a fee regularly, even when not using their services.]

'It's all got to come in the right order. There's no point getting stressed out about getting a lawyer or manager or agent. What you have to do before you get into any of that stuff is create a personality with which people want to engage. It has to be memorable; the songs, how you play, how you look and how you behave. All the elements have to come together and be convincing. Once you've got that right people will start taking notice and that's when you need to think about a lawyer.'

How long did you spend in the studio and was the budget enough?
'We spent a total of around 30 days recording and mixing the album, in various studios. To keep the overall time down, we rehearsed like hell before we got into any kind of studio.

'Money just disappears when you're recording. We were using other people's money and it was important to spend it as carefully as possible. The overspend was caused by our underestimation of how long it would take to get things right in the studio.

'This is really important: before you set foot in the studio you must be able to play all your music backwards, forwards and sideways without mistakes. You have to know what you want from a song. Obviously, mistakes will happen – but be careful. It's the songs that haven't been gigged that cause trouble.'

Learning from experience, Clear advise the following if you are recording in a studio and paying top dollar by the hour.

- Spend the money where it's best spent – on drums and vocals.

- Only hire a 'good' studio for drums (found by word of mouth) because drums make the difference between a good record and a bad record. Spend the money and get the perfection here, then everything else is easily layered on top. Most other things you can record in your bedroom.

- You will need extra budget for editing.

- It's really important to find an experienced producer whom you can trust: they'll protect you from a lot of rubbish and you'll learn a lot from them.

- Save money by practising before the studio is booked.

CASH AND BLING

The digital age is renewing and refreshing the industry and, at the same time, blasting dusty relics out of the arena. Singles sales are doing well after seeming to collapse a couple of years ago; and album sales are struggling after some analysts thought that they were invincible.

'The arrival of digital retail has restored the singles market to its 1990s high in just two years. That British signed and developed acts are also taking a growing slice of an album market is something to celebrate; clearly the record industry is adapting successfully to change.'

www.brits.co.uk

FASCINATING FACT

UK record companies invest proportionately more in research and development than the aerospace and defence industries, the car industry and even the computer industry.
Source: **British Recorded Music Industry (BPI)**

How can you strike gold? Where is the money? According to the BPI (British Phonographic Industry), yearly album sales top £200 million and have done since the mid-1990s but profits are down because of deals and price cutting in the high street. It looks like the industry is pulling one way and retailing is pulling the other.

Post-teenagers, who are thought to have disposable income (money left after all the bills are paid), dominate the album-buying world. Teenagers are thought to have less spending power and are said to dominate the single-buying public.

The singles chart is the catwalk of the music industry, introducing the listener to the artist, and gives easy access to impulse shopping.

There are hundreds of articles on whether those who download illegally from the internet are a threat to the music business or not. Some say the industry profits because those same people then go out to the shops to buy the album. There's no question, though, that the industry will hit back with expensive legal cases. In the US, university students are finding this out to their cost via some very high-profile cases.

However, it will always be the case that people still love to acquire music. A lot of our personality is expressed through our music preference. Perhaps it is very primal that we have to have a personal music collection that reflects who we are.

SALES: HOW TO STRIKE GOLD

● How many CDs can a new artist expect to sell?

● How many CDs will a record company manufacture?

According to Donald Passman's book, *All You Need To Know About the Music Business*, a new artist is someone who hasn't sold over 250,000 albums.

The box below gives the figures for achieving Silver, Gold and Platinum sales for albums and singles, as set out by the IFPI (International Federation of Phonographic Industries, www.ifpi.org).

ALBUM AND SINGLE SALES

Albums: Silver = 60,000
Gold = 100,000
Platinum = 300,000
Double Platinum = 600,000

Singles: Silver = 200,000
Gold = 400,000
Platinum = 600,000
Double Platinum = 1.2 million

To put these figures into context, the first album by the Arctic Monkeys (*Whatever They Say I Am, I'm Not*) holds the record for the fastest-selling British debut album with 364,000 copies sold in the first week, which is immediate Platinum. According to the band's website their second album (*Favourite Worst Nightmare*) sold 85,000 copies on its first day of sale. The album went straight into the charts at No 1 and also renewed interest in the previous album.

CHAPTER 4

Recording and producing

THE RECORDING STUDIO

A recording studio is a thing of beauty. The ultimate recording studio can be found at number 3 Abbey Road – the most famous recording studio in the world. It is home to not only the most famous Beatles recordings but also to classical music and music hall favourites, film soundtracks and artists, from Fred Astaire and Paul Robeson to Robbie Williams, Muse and Baaba Maal.

It is impossible to pick out a few names and do justice to the variety of legends and megastars that have enjoyed the facilities. The studio opened in 1931 and the weight of history in the atmosphere is overwhelming. Take a look at the full history of recording from the days of Sir Edward Elgar to today: www.abbeyroad.co.uk.

Since 2005 the newest British bands have piled into the studio for one week in February to enjoy the happy ghosts of Studio 2 where the Beatles recorded. Established artists mix with newcomers: 2007 saw over 30 bands including Katie Melua, Simon Webb and The Dualers play sets broadcast to over 130 countries. Breakfast show host Ted Kelly's enthusiasm for British music drives the project to a yearly celebration of new, established and unsigned bands. I'm lucky enough to be his co-host and to interview the artists.

A whole week of *UPOP Sessions @ Abbey Road* are broadcast on a host of platforms (which gives an indication of how the music industry is changing out of all recognition): Worldspace Satellite Radio, XM, AOL, DirecTV and Napster. Another sign of change is how the consumer can buy session music, not just finite, contained and studio-produced tunes.

Could your band be on the line-up in the next year?

There are many other recording studios that have their own magic and history. The next two profiles give an insight into the recording studio and the engineering needs of the studio. After these examples there are profiles of two producers.

'We can't give work experience to anyone who doesn't have the technical basics. Why would we give a job as a runner to someone to just make tea for the artists? There's no point. They must want to progress and to have the means of doing that.'

Andrea Terrano, Iguana Studios

Big studios are sponsored by major labels (like the Hollywood studio system of yesteryear). The artists are in place and have proven themselves as big sellers, the facilities are in place, the mechanics of making the finished product are in place, the legal and financial systems are by and large dictated by the big companies and the finished product is assured to a certain standard for a certain market. It all works like clockwork.

This is the traditional, conservative, status quo end of the studio spectrum. Record company artists are fed through their own collection of studios. Abbey Road studios, for example, is one of the studios owned by EMI.

According to Andrea Terrano, if you want to be a 'pure' engineer, this role really only exists in the record companies' studios. To get work in a studio you could offer yourself as a runner, from where you can hope to work your way up from tea maker, to tape operator, to assistant ... and this is where you start getting credit and really being involved.

ANDREA TERRANO, IGUANA STUDIOS

Now the proud owner of Iguana Studios in Brixton, Andrea Terrano's career path has included: being in a band, studying sound engineering, teaching, and finally selling his flat to build a dream studio. With no financial backing, the studio was built brick by brick with the help of friends and contacts that he made through his time in the industry. For Andrea there is nothing as important as being diplomatic and making good contacts. Without his friends and contacts, his studio couldn't have been built.

According to Andrea, the first thing you must know is that every engineer is also a programmer. The competition is tough and you must be able to program on the major software platforms as a basic skill to offer the employer.

The box below lists the major software platforms. Andrea's website lists the software his studio offers to clients: Audio Logic 6.4, ProTools LE, Wavebourner Pro, Emagic and Powercore pluggings (see www.iguanastudio.co.uk).

Terrano Tips

- 'If you are able to say that you are familiar with Logic it shows that you are ready for a job with a studio. The demand is huge for someone who knows what they are doing.'

- 'You must be able to offer a good CV. Don't make it too colourful but don't make it dull.'

- You need luck. Andrea says: 'Be in the right place at the right time!'.

Background

Andrea is a musician who is also a sound engineer. He says that when you add these two together you get a producer.

Andrea came from Italy to study English and sound engineering at the School of Audio Engineering (SAE). This venture was supported by his parents. He doesn't know if it would have been possible without them. This is important to him as a great motivating force. When you finally make the break, 'it proves to your parents that they were right to put their faith in you'.

At the same time he studied composition, took Grade 5 music theory and took harmony classes. 'In that sense, living in a city is ideal because of the access you have to short courses.' Never underestimate the power of the teacher to be an industry contact. The composition teacher at Goldsmiths helped Andrea to get a teaching job at Music Works (now Raw Materials) in Brixton.

As a teacher at Music Works, Andrea took the chance to make a useful contact. He arranged to take his class in a studio rather than in the college environment. He did some research, found a studio and introduced himself. He chose one that was still using the analogue system: it was the old-school way of working with tape, not with computers.

Working in this studio, Andrea savoured the last of the pre-digital world and learnt everything he could about analogue and tape, quite apart from being surrounded by history and people talking about having worked with Bob Marley. It was the last echoes of an era. You can see how Andrea would be so inspired to own a studio.

At the same time, Andrea was slowly buying equipment for his home studio. Eventually, he had a complete studio in his living room, where his clientele and confidence grew. This is the beginning of the process that saw him sell his flat and build his studio. He found a shell of a building and had enough vision and enough money for the task – and a sympathetic girlfriend willing to give him a home!

Terrano Tip
You may have already decided against formal training and formal qualifications, but a teacher may help you to make contacts and to network, and may even be your access to your first break.

Iguana Studios

With his new studio ready for business, Andrea needed to find some clients. His strategy was to advertise in *Loot*. You have to phone the newspaper to find out their rates but Andrea paid £500 for three months. This worked as far as getting in the first few clients. Since then, Andrea has built his corporate client list to include BMG, EMI, the BBC, Sony Publishing, Lion Music, Young Money Records and the Ministry of Sound.

As Managing Director, Andrea now employs five staff (producers, engineers and programmers, as well as information technology and website design people). Iguana also has a long list of bands and singers.

Terrano Tip
Keep organised accounting records. When you need to go to the bank to ask for a business loan, you need to prove that you are capable of bringing in work and running a professional business concern. Without a track record, how will a bank know what to make of you?

Words of advice

- Don't give up!

- Repay the work of your teachers and the faith of your parents.

- If you know how to use Logic, send Andrea your CV!

MAJOR SOFTWARE PLATFORMS FOR RECORDING

- Cubase VST/SX (newsrooms use a variety of editing packages including DALET, but as long as you have a basic understanding of editing skills, even Garageband or a similar music editing package, then these skills can be updated and transferred)

- Logic Audio (Andrea Terrano recommends Logic but hard-disk editing on software such as SADiE and Adobe Audition will give transferable skills)

- Pro Tools

- Sona.

Ensure that you understand both Mac and PC platforms. It is especially important not to restrict yourself to one or the other, but to have a basic knowledge of both operating systems.

Here is a description of Cubase (www.cubase.com):

Cubase is a complete virtual studio with a tape recorder, a mixer, effects processors and electronic instruments all in one integrated space. It is an audio editing and sequencing 'environment'. Cubase VST has largely been replaced by the newer SX. VST has a lot of faithful users but SX includes a technology called System Link that allows you to use more than one computer at a time.

CAREER OPTIONS

Here are some of the job titles in recording and producing roles:

- **assistant engineer**: an entry point to a recording career

- **engineer**: operates the mixing console and works with all technical aspects of recording and production of audio

- **producer**: works with record labels, artists/bands and composers to oversee all aspects of production: ultimately, the producer has to make recordings that are marketable

- **sound editor**: found in the film industry, this is the creative person behind the soundtrack; edits effects, dialogue and music

- **sound engineer**: sets up the studio, positions the performers' equipment, monitors sound levels and dynamics, records each instrument, mixes different tracks on tape, and compiles the recordings into the final master

- **studio manager**: responsible for all aspects of the recording studio, this person needs excellent management skills, financial know-how and knowledge of the technical and creative aspects of music production – credibility with clients depends on this (see the profile of Andrea Terrano on pages 34–36).

SOUND ENGINEER

Neil Gardener is a teacher at the Gateway School of Recording and Music Technology at Kingston University (www.gsr.org.uk), which is a centre for education and training in sound engineering, music production, multimedia and the music industry. He summarises the role of the sound engineer in the box below.

'Sound engineers make mammoth contributions to the overall feel of a track. They may not get the big name recognition of producers, but without them the recorded music wouldn't exist.'

Neil Gardener, Gateway School of Recording and Music Technology

NEIL GARDENER, GATEWAY SCHOOL OF RECORDING AND MUSIC TECHNOLOGY

What should we know about 'soundies'?

'They are full of gossip and insight about the superstars they work with, but very honest, trustworthy and circumspect in professional circles. You never find exposés and revelations in tabloids because of a soundie. Their motivation is entirely different.'

What does a sound engineer actually do?

'Well, it's a complicated answer, because sound engineers do a lot, and many of them do a lot in a lot of different areas of the music industry. Every album, single, piece of music on television, radio or the internet – in fact, everything you hear that is not live has been recorded by a sound engineer. This is no easy job.

'You need a great pair of ears (and you must protect them – so no more standing next to the speakers in clubs, or listening through your headphones at full volume!). You need to love and understand music. You need an interest in the technical side of music and you need to be a great people manager.

'In among all these things, you need to be able to record the live output of a band or musician and then reproduce it off tape, CD or computer in a way that doesn't misrepresent the artist's work. In essence, it is the sound engineer who takes the music from the musician and passes it along to the listener.'

How does a sound engineer do all these things?

'Like most professions it comes with a lot of training and even more practice. The sound engineer must be able to control a recording studio confidently – everything from microphone selection and placement, through to the understanding of acoustics and reverberation, the control of a multi-channel mixing console, and the use of EQ, reverb, echo, distortion, and a host of other exciting sound-manipulation tools.

'The sound engineer also needs to understand the process of mixing different sounds together. Here is where you can specialise, as there are many sound engineers who only do recording, and those that only do the final mixing. The final mix of an album or track can make it or break it, so this is generally another step up in the art of the professional sound engineer: your career progresses to sound mixer.

'Finally, the sound engineer needs to be able to set up and run the recording technology, be it for 2" master tapes, recordable CDs or via hard-disk systems and external hard drives.'

What are the downsides?
The sound engineer needs to be a diplomat. There's nothing more complex than the relationships between the musicians, their friends, colleagues and music-business types. A recording session can quickly become a tangled web of egos and arguments.

'Then there's the constant repetition, of lyrics, drum loops, guitar breaks, etc. You think you like music? Some might say there's nothing worse than hearing the same 20 seconds of a song a hundred times, day in, day out, and having to wait while the artists work out how to get it just right. On the other hand, that's where the passion for the job kicks in.

'And then there's the hours. Creating music is a difficult and time-consuming process that can go on for months. And when someone gets 'in the groove' the sound engineer can't turn around and say: "But it's 6pm, I've gotta go home now".'

Is sound engineering a good career?
'I have to say yes, it is, because I love recording, mixing and mastering. There's a thrill to knowing that you're the person who made the music accessible to millions of listeners. There's the thrill of being at the recording and experiencing the creation of new music and knowing that it was your technical and creative decisions that contributed to the final sound.

'The best musicians recognise the value of a good sound engineer and usually work with the same people year after year. This applies as much for live-sound engineers, final-mix engineers and the specialist-genre engineers (classical or jazz). It may not pay the most money, but you'll never go hungry.'

How can I become a sound engineer?

'Courses allow you to spend time in real studios, recording real bands under the guidance of professional and active sound engineers. You also learn about music-business law, surround-sound mixing, live sound, hard-disk editing and sound for vision and Mml (mobile mark-up language) technologies.

'More and more, professional studios are seeking out young engineers with these qualifications, rather than taking on people who may be enthusiastic but lack hands-on experience.'

If you're getting excited and shouting 'I want to have a go!', then you are perfect sound-engineer material. Why? Because sound engineering is a passion and a vocation. A 4-minute song can take days or even weeks to record. You can easily spend a whole day just setting the microphones for a drum kit! And there's no slacking. If the artist wants to record through the night, then that's what you do.

If you want to become a sound engineer you should:

● read sound engineering magazines such as *Sound On Sound* and *Pro Sound*

● read as many sound-engineering books as you can find

● get involved with the live sound at a local club or live venue

● listen to a lot of different styles of music and analyse them; work out how they were made

● invest some time and money in getting qualified.

'For the engineer it's not so much sex, drugs and rock 'n' roll, but decks, mugs of tea and sausage rolls! In all this, the sound engineer is in the middle of things, ensuring everything works, sounds good and is being recorded. Without the sound engineer nothing would happen.'

Neil Gardener, Gateway School of Recording and Music Technology

---

JARGON BOX

EQ: equalisation for correction and sound enhancement in the wake of distortion.

Reverb: a reflected signal, as if in a cave. The quality of each sound is different and, unlike a delay, it is a diffuse, continuously smooth decay of sound.

Echo: the reflection of sound from a surface such as a wall or a floor; a distinct, recognisable repetition (or series of repetitions) of a word, note, phrase or sound.

PRODUCER

The following is a list of famous producers, and the artists who have worked with them:

- Dr. Dre: Snoop Dogg, Eminem, 50 Cent

- Missy Elliott: Whitney Houston, Janet Jackson, Christina Aguilera, Justin Timberlake, Destiny's Child

- Trevor Horn: Lisa Stansfield, Frankie Goes To Hollywood, Grace Jones, Seal

- Sir George Martin: The Beatles (sometimes called 'The Fifth Beatle')

- Tony Visconti: T.Rex, Iggy Pop, David Bowie, U2.

But what does a producer actually do? The following two profiles explore the role of the producer. Ahmad Dayes explains how he got into producing; and Tai Newsam (aka Shredda) tells us how to roll up our sleeves and do it ourselves.

'Once you get into the realm of putting your ideas down, you are producing.'

Ahmad Dayes, Producer

AHMAD DAYES, PRODUCER
Ahmad Dayes is a producer who creates backing tracks for vocalists. He runs the recording sessions and also mixes the tracks. He has been producing since he was 18 years old. For five years now he has been producing a variety of genres from hip hop, r'n'b, and drum and bass, to more party-orientated tracks.

Ahmad is always trying to create the next new sound. He draws on his classical training, which he acquired through playing in orchestras and symphonic bands in his childhood. He plays the trombone and the piano, which have proven to be a great source of inspiration. His ambition is to break through to the mainstream and set up his own record label.

'The reason that I got into producing and engineering was in order to make drum and bass music. It's not a genre of music that is possible to create without using some sort of music technology.

'I had a brief encounter with Cubase when I was at school so I had a very vague idea of how it might be possible to start making tunes. I was lucky enough to meet someone who made drum and bass. Through regular visits I started to pick up the process of putting a tune together.

'The next stage for me was to start training myself in the skills needed to operate a studio. The first – and still one of the most important – things I had to learn was how to operate a computer with music software. I enrolled on an evening Cubase course which taught me how to put my ideas down. Once you get into the realm of putting your ideas down, you are producing.

'I found that the learning curve got quite steep once I was making tunes and taking them away to work on them again. Your ears start to develop a taste for sounds and rhythms quite fast. But one thing that I remember doing a lot more was listening to other people's music and working out how they put their tunes together.

'If I was really going to make tunes seriously I would need some equipment to get me started. Strategically the one piece of equipment that was really going to help me would be a computer. Ever since I had my own computer I have been able to make music when I want and how I want. When that special idea comes around and you get it down, you know what it's all about.

'My next move was to enrol on a course at the Midi Music Company (MMC: www.themidimusiccompany.co.uk), which looked at the creative aspect of making music at the same time as the technical side. Being on that course really opened up my mind as I started getting experience working with, and for, other people. I enrolled on other courses that went further into the studio side of the process. After that I was asked to help out and do a bit of vocal recording for another course that was going on.

'I felt like I had been thrust into the deep end but that is the fastest way to learn. Being involved at MMC has given me a base from which to work. I started to make music for vocalists of different styles and found that they brought something to my music that I couldn't get when making purely instrumental tracks.

'One of the ways that I work is to give vocalists a selection of ideas on a CD to pick over. When they have got comfortable with that idea and have written something for it, we lay it down on computer. This really enables me to get into the tune more. It creates the bigger picture.

'Being involved with MMC has been a good support. One of the reasons I was able to get free studio time was that I did a lot of volunteering for them and looked after the equipment. Plus MMC is an organisation set up to help young people get involved in the music game.

'Through working with other people and trying out new ideas you pick up the skills faster. As an independent producer you have to be an engineer as well as a producer. The two go hand in hand because if you can engineer you can save a hell of a lot of time and money creating a finished piece of music.

'As inspiration is somewhat of a random thing, it is very important to be able to get ideas down when they come to you. If you don't have the skills to put an idea down when you get it, you lose it. It's strange that there are infinite possibilities with music, yet you can go weeks without getting that spark. Even when you do get that spark, it can seem impossible to finish the tune.

'Through putting yourself through the motions you pick up all the details that count. By making yourself available to work on a regular basis you learn much faster and get more comfortable with your working environment.

'You can't expect to learn the theory and then be able to go out and make a living from it. Experience, experience, experience is what gets you where you want to be, so you've got to grab and make opportunities for yourself to gain that experience.

'Everyone has their own way of doing things. It's about finding yours and constantly adjusting it to work in all situations.'

FASCINATING FACT

Bob Ezrin was a teenager when he started producing records for other teenagers. That was in the early 1970s. At 19 years old he co-produced Alice Cooper's entire debut album, *Love It To Death*. Later, he rearranged Pink Floyd's 'Another Brick in the Wall (Part II)' into an accessible hit-single format. He had an immense knowledge of music theory but his teenage gift was that he was more versatile than the pop producers of the day and he rebelled against the recording standards of the day.

Source: **emusician.com**

TAI NEWSAM, SHREDDA PRODUCTIONS

Tai Newsam (aka Shredda) first started producing when he was 14 years old, and is now 16 years old. He attended Gladesmore Community School, which is a school in Tottenham where he was able to practise producing different types of music such as rap, hip hop and garage (which is now known as grime). As a producer he has organised studio time for artists and produced many backing tracks for vocalists. He has created a new genre that is generated by different styles of music and he calls this genre 'waterful muezick'. Tai's music sounds very adventurous, which may mirror his joy when playing computer games. His main ambition is to achieve worldwide recognition of his new genre and to have his own record label. You can find out more about Shredda on www.myspace.com/shreddaproductionz.

The start

I started producing on a program called Reason 1.5 (see p48 for a screenshot) which is owned by the company Propellerhead. As I began to use this program I had no clue what I was doing because all I saw were a lot of buttons and machines so I decided to get somebody who has experience with this program to teach me the basics. I got an older student to stay with me in the music room after school hours. After a few lessons I finally learned the basics.

'I became a producer because most of the people around me were into music so I quickly got attached to it.'

Influences

'My main influence is computer games. While playing on Playstation One I used to listen to a lot of the soundtrack music that had been used for battles and travelling. Therefore, if you listen to my instrumentals you will be able to realise that they could be used not just for rap, hip hop and grime, but also for film soundtracks and computer games. Also, I have been influenced by rap and hip hop producers such as Scott Scorch, Timberland and Neptunes.'

The way forward

'At 15 years old I took a music course in my school which would teach me the basics of producing music. Mr Parker was the first teacher to show me about Reason. The support I got from this course was helpful: the teacher would give me a beat he had made and would ask me to make the same beat but a different version of it. For example, if his beat was jazz, I would have to make a rap version. Also, he would give me homework sheets, asking me questions about the machines that hold the instruments, how I create a loop and how I copy and paste. Importantly, the good thing about taking the course was that it taught at a tempo that was suitable for me.

'As a producer I had to learn many skills to help perfect my talent, like the keys on a piano. It's one of the first things you need to learn because, while using a music program such as Reason and Cubase, a piano is used for almost every instrument except for the drum patterns. The advantage of using Reason is that you don't have to play the piano to make a beat; you can use the attachable keyboard on the screen to draw in your melody and bass.

'My theory is that anybody can be a producer. As long as you work hard and focus, you can achieve anything. Practise, practise, practise is all you need.'

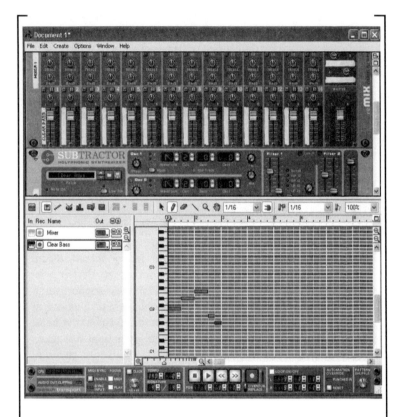

Equipment helps

'There is so much equipment that will help your music tremendously. I advise you to purchase a MIDI keyboard, powerful speakers, a microphone condenser and a mixer.

'These are just examples of what is good to use but if you can't purchase all of them, just try to get good speakers. I personally only have good speakers at home because I feel I don't need all of those things at the moment.'

Music programs

'Reason 3.0, Fruity Loops Studio, Cubase and Logic are the music programs I recommend. To start off, I would suggest you use Fruity Loops because it is the most basic program to learn quickly. Then I would move on to Cubase because I believe it is an easy program to adapt to even though it is slightly harder than FL Studio.

'When you know you can produce a basic beat and can use Cubase, then I feel you are ready to use Reason, which is not hard to learn if you have somebody teaching you. However, it is hard to make professional sounds: for top quality, you will need to learn how to mix your tunes.

'Finally, you should be able to produce a full instrumental, including a drum pattern, melody and bass. At this stage you should be ready to use Logic. I advise this program last because it is very difficult to use.'

Independent producing
'Working as an independent producer is difficult in some ways, such as pushing my tracks forward, because not being in a crew [group] means I have less connection to other producers and managers. However, my hard work and inspiration meant that I was able to get in contact with some producers so that I started to do joint productions.

'As an independent producer, I had to find a quick way to promote my music so I signed up for a Hotmail account. This was useful because I could then talk on MSN Messenger, which helps me to get in contact with other artists. Also, if I enjoy a person's music on MySpace, I can give them my Hotmail address for email contact.

'After college I'll make beats probably five days a week. As I kept getting more positive comments about my work, and more promotion, I then got recognised by an organisation called New Era, which is a team that help each other to fulfil their dream by working on tracks together to show the listeners that we do serious music.

'My advice to other independent producers is to stay focused and take in constructive criticism because it will drive you to the next level and then you will only get better and better. Listen to other people's music for inspiration because you will always learn from others. Always look for opportunities, but think before you take because you don't want to join a record label that's not right for you. Also, remember you have your own style that's unique, so never feel the music you make is not right because as long as there's an instrument then it's music.'

CHAPTER 5

Work experience

WHY DO I NEED WORK EXPERIENCE?

It is important to get work experience for so many reasons. It gives you a flavour of the workplace and an insight into the industry. You get hands-on experience as well as a chance to shine and to impress people. You get to know yourself and if the music industry is the right career choice for you. There is the possibility of 'getting your foot in the door' and making contacts that will be useful later. Ultimately, work experience will build up your CV: it shows you to be actively and genuinely interested in getting a job in the industry.

Work experience allows you to go to an employer and have a very clear idea of what you have to offer. If you are leaving school or university, then work experience is an excellent use of your time.

Perhaps you will be offered a job after your work experience, but if you aren't, then it's possible that they weren't convinced about where you would fit in and you haven't made a very strong case. Don't worry, stay focused, and don't get bogged down with taking rejection personally.

To make the most of your work experience, you should consider the following questions before you start at a company.

- Where will you be placed in the company?

- Is it a platform from which you can learn about the company?

- Will colleagues get to know you and will you get an opportunity to shine?

- What have you got to offer? Do you have a unique selling point?

- Can you make an unpromising job an opportunity to cultivate contacts?

- Can you make the most positive use of your time in the company?

- Who in the company can you ask for help and direction?

- You are working for free for a clear reason. What is that reason?

'I think I got on really well with the people, I was willing to try really hard at even the most boring job they could offer and still have a laugh with everyone. I would go to any gig that had spare tickets which meant I got to talk to people outside the office environment: quite often I could chat and have a few beers with the MD [managing director] of Sony International; time and advice I never would have got during office hours.'

Sam Eldridge, Band Manager

WHAT CAN I LEARN FROM WORK EXPERIENCE?

Your school may send you to a record company and you'll have to cope for a week or two in the office environment, where people are likely to be too busy to take your fledgling career by the hand and lead you into the big time. You could call up and ask for some kind of job description to prepare yourself, but companies might just be too busy. In reality, they will want you to run around, send out mail and generally make yourself useful.

This may not excite you but you will be in the privileged position of being on the inside, and seeing how a company works. In conversations that fly back and forth you'll hear what kind of knowledge people have about the industry, and you'll hear their telephone conversations and their negotiations. Make notes. Ask questions.

To prepare for work experience, do some homework: find out about the company, their clientele, their successes, recent achievements, and their structure. This is the minimum homework to be done. It is a mistake to go for a job placement without having found out about the company. This won't impress anyone. You need to make it clear to colleagues that you are genuinely interested. Basic homework is one way of doing that.

Don't be daunted. Dive in. Have a go.

AN EXAMPLE OF WORK EXPERIENCE

Anglo Plugging (www.angloplugging.co.uk) is an independent promotion and management company that is in the habit of offering work experience. Providing national and regional radio, television and online promotion, Anglo claims that, by using their services, the artist is buying time, contacts and expertise. Whether an artist is looking for their first radio play or is about to embark on a fifth album launch, Anglo forms a strategy with artist management, press agents and record companies to assess the areas of exposure. They select the best release dates and timing of events and use computer tracking to list all radio-station plays.

A 'plugger' is a music promoter who is hired by a record company to 'plug' or sell music to radio stations and television companies. It is a job that depends on good relationships with contacts in the radio and television industries. A good record promoter needs good social skills, enthusiasm and persistence. You need connections at both the labels (to get hired) and the radio and television stations (to get results).

Alice Schofield is from Anglo Plugging and she gives her thoughts on work experience in the box below.

ALICE SCHOFIELD, ANGLO PLUGGING
Do you have an example of a typical work experience candidate?
'We had a girl called Sasha in for work experience one week. She was 16 years old, doing her GCSEs, not necessarily planning on being in the music industry but was keen to learn all the same. She was friendly, chatty and, above all, helpful. You could always rely on her to do any job for you no matter how menial it was. She really fitted in as part of the team and it was just a shame we had to let her go at the end of the week.'

What is the key to a successful experience?
'The best advice I can give is to be proactive. Never sit there with nothing to do; always ask around if there's anything you can do to help. Always be prepared to do menial tasks and carry them out to your best ability; never show you are bored or unhappy with any task you've been given; always come across as happy to help.

'Asking questions is the best way to learn, but the pupil must also realise that we have a job to do, so they can't be asking questions all day! I've always been impressed with pupils that are keen to know exactly what we do, and how to go about getting into this job.'

What jobs always need doing?
'Stickering up and mailing out CDs and records. A work experience person will mainly be helping with mail-outs as this is the bulk of our job. Other tasks they may be given are things such as typing up press releases and tour dates. And, of course, there's filing.'

Who is the work experience likely to be with? Marketing? Plugging?
'They will work with the plugging team. No chances to go out to radio stations unfortunately, but if we are doing an event they may be asked to come and help out there.'

What should a candidate not do? What behaviour and attitude will not impress?
'There was a guy who asked if he could come in for work experience. Before he started he was told that we wouldn't pay any expenses and that the main work would be mailing out records. When he came he kicked up a fuss and was rude, left after two days and then wrote an email to our head of promotions complaining. We replied that had he stuck it out he would have found that he would have been given more things to do, plus he should realise that in every job you need to start at the bottom; nothing should be below you.

'He left us with a very sour taste in our mouths and I am very careful now about the people I take on. I make sure that they know they will be doing a lot of menial tasks. This does not mean that these tasks are not an important part of learning about the job. The best way to learn is to start at the bottom and work your way up. You need to learn about the job by asking questions and seeing how others work.

'Another example of someone who didn't impress was a girl who came in and didn't say a word for the whole week; never came up and asked for things to do. She would just sit there reading a magazine until you asked her to do a job. When she'd finished she wouldn't say "I've finished", but would just go back to reading the magazine.

'A work experience person should be more proactive. I like a work experience person to enjoy their time here, but it really is a lot to do with them and how they approach the job. A happy, smiley and chatty person is likely to get along much better than someone who's quiet and unconfident.

> 'A work experience person should make the most out of their week by asking questions and being proactive; always be prepared for doing boring jobs!'

According to Alice, the important issues to learn about work experience are that the work will probably be 'menial' and 'boring' because you are starting at the bottom. Alice has seen work experience people who were disappointed with their time and so she wants to make it clear that you won't be running the company in your first week. Nevertheless, you have to impress. You are finding out about the world of work.

WORK ETIQUETTE

Here are things you must do in all walks of life from nine to five:

- always be on time: lateness is not impressive

- always employ manners: knock on doors before entering, say 'excuse me' if you urgently have to interrupt a conversation, or 'sorry to bother you but . . .' if you're asking for help or another task. Do your best not to interrupt conversations

- you could offer to get a round of coffees for your colleagues

- greet people properly in the morning and make sure when you leave that you haven't left undone work or an untidy desk

- always be polite to colleagues, from the receptionist in the morning to the late-night cleaners.

These are basic qualities that everyone – at any age and in any job – should observe.

CHAPTER 6

Job profiles of coveted careers

CAREER ADVICE

This chapter has advice from a selection of professionals who have made it into successful careers: artist manager, marketing manager, DJ/artist, manager at a live-music venue and festival organiser.

These professionals offer guidance, recommendations and descriptions of their own experiences of starting out that will help you form a picture of what your career path may look like. They have practical advice to give, and a go-out-and-do-it attitude that should rouse your desire.

ARTIST MANAGER

Chapter 2 included a list of some of the most popular jobs in the music industry (see page 15). Artist manager features on this list and is deemed to be a sexy spot for the whizz organiser. This chapter gives the profile of Sam Eldridge, and he gives the impression that he was an intern one week and a band manager the next. His story has a lot of confidence to it.

Refer to the British Phonographic Industry (BPI) website once again for the maps and flow charts showing the industry structure (www.bpi-med.co.uk). Click on 'artist management' and you will see that it is the manager who stands between the artist and recording, performing, publishing and promotion. The map indicates that the manager of an artist has to be in contact with dozens of elements of the industry, so that they can take care of the business side, and the day-to-day realities, of the artists' careers.

When researching managers of bands a few common themes emerge. Many managers seem to know key members of a band from school and get roped in to doing all the jobs other than music making. This is a happy accident if managing a band is your goal.

'Create a following and a story. Things that would contribute to a story would be various data that we could track – sold-out shows, record sales, and getting airplay on their own. That happens all the time. Those are things that virtually all A&R people look for.'
Tom Sarig, Vice President of A&R, MCA Records

SAM ELDRIDGE, BAND MANAGER
Sam Eldridge is the manager of Ludes, an r'n'b outfit.

How did you meet Ludes? Is it ever a problem that you are friends?
'Managing Ludes was a kind of great accident, like a lot of things in music. I knew the guitarist James and just thought it would be good to have something of my own outside of my job at Sony. I started doing it part time until it became a full-time job, and it turned into a career when we got our deals and started earning a bit of money as well.

'You can get too close to an act and lose some vital critical distance, or if you are mates to start with you might fall out over the sometimes harsh realities you have to give the band.

The best thing is to keep some distance and separate the biz side with the mates side and, as long as everyone is clear where that line is, all should be cool.

'But don't expect it to happen overnight. Quite often the biggest bands have been quietly slogging away for years before anyone hears a note.'

What does a manager do?
'It's a case of encouraging them creatively and putting them at the right venues at the right time. There are loads of clubs in London where all the A&R [artist and repertoire] guys go (they tend to hunt in packs), but a manager has to choose the right time to go there. You have to be confident that you have created a following and that the band's material is as strong as it could be.'

Where did you learn how to build up a fan base and how to build a strategy?
'During my time at the Sony press office, I got a great insight into why some bands capture the public's imagination and others just don't. This led me to want to work in A&R where you actually find those bands and work with them on the creative side. A&R really opened my eyes as to what a band needs to achieve in terms of plot and strategy to become successful and get signed.'

Who is in your team and where did they come from?
'As well as A&R people you will often find independent press and promotion people, as well as agents, at the right gigs. These people will sometimes offer to work for free at first so that they can be involved when the band "breaks".

'There are quite a lot of independent press and promotions people around and it's a question of research: which artists do they represent; would you like to be associated with those artists; and has the PR [Public Relations] and marketing worked well for them?

'Once you have your team (press – getting you in the magazines; promotion – pushing you to radio and television; agent – booking your gigs), the manager's job is to co-ordinate all these aspects so that they are all driving towards the same point at the right time, generally around a single or album release.

'Aside from this you have a lawyer and an accountant who can be instrumental in getting you the right deal and pushing you to the best people; again they will often hang out at key venues in order to pick up bands.'

Is it always best to sign with a big company?
'Generally the bigger companies have more power and so can push your band into the right areas. However, small companies may treat you as a priority and work even harder for you. I guess it's all a question of what fits the band.'

How do you build up a fan base?
'We have street teams of young kids in each town who hand out flyers, get emails from fans, and generally raise awareness of the band in their town. This can be a great way for young people interested in the music business to get some contact with people at record companies.

'To build up a local fan base try and do something original that sets you apart from the crowd. There's no real point touring till you have some sort of press coverage, radio play and a fan base.'

How do you organise a tour?
'Our tour was booked through an agent, who knows what size venues we can fill according to the band's profile. The tour was quite heavily supported by Xfm [a London radio station] and *NME*, which guarantees some support.'

What are the pitfalls and rewards of being a manager?
'It can take over your life. It's not a nine-to-five job. I have recently taken on a couple of new acts, moved to a new office

and I'm looking to set up a studio with my partner. It's all a case of building slowly but surely, and in a business where there are no set rules. I was an intern one week and a manager the next. It's a case of going for every opportunity, no matter how small it may seem.'

The music press are all in a tizz about the changing nature of the biz. Are you?
'The internet has had a massive effect on the music business and my job is to react positively to this, be it with downloadable singles, ringtones or whatever. Like everything else, as a manager you've got to see how best you can rig it to your band's advantage.'

FASCINATING FACT

Elton John famously rang up his management office one day to complain about the wind blowing noisily outside his window and demanding that they do something about it.

Brian Ferry allegedly tore up his passport on the eve of an American visit because he quite simply didn't like the look of his passport photograph.
Source: **Paul Charles,** *The Complete Guide to Playing Live*

MARKETING MANAGER

Marketing and promotions is a much sought-after position. It is a job that gets you involved with the artist, in their recordings, performances and video shoots, as well as constant interaction with the press.

Since he arrived in the UK in the mid 1990s, Oliver X has spent time in various jobs outside of the music industry. He finally broke through and got a marketing manager job with a major label before becoming a freelance artist manager. He is now Head Buyer with an international music distribution company and is based in Barcelona. In this job, he buys CDs from all over the world so that they can be distributed in Spain, negotiating prices and conditions of payment. He also listens to a lot of new music so that he can choose relevant titles. The job takes him to many cities to meet with record companies. The box below follows his career path.

OLIVER X, MARKETING MANAGER

The marketing department of a record company is *the* cool place to be. Oliver lives a life of wild European travel and after-show parties. He mixes with artists and gets loads of free CDs. He always has lovely clothes and great haircuts. He discovers and frequents the best venues. I want to be him! I asked him how to do that. I discovered that it would take planning, focus, patience and buckets of motivation, as well as money for countless phone calls.

First he studied marketing and business techniques in his degree (a BSc in European Business and Technology), before studying for a master's degree in Sales and Marketing from the University of Montpellier in France. During his studies, he lived in France, Spain and the UK. His mother tongue is French but he moved around to improve his languages. He had finished his studies by the time he was 22 years old.

He worked in a medical equipment company after graduating but was a DJ at parties and weddings and spent his spare time reading all the music weeklies and magazines. He was always looking for contacts in the radio and music industry and when he was 23 years old, he sent CVs to Paris, London, Madrid and Barcelona, where he knew music scenes existed and were active.

He chased up every CV with phone calls – but nobody returned his calls! All the companies sent back rejection letters. Finally, he got through to somebody at a radio production company in London who suggested he come to London for a meeting, without making any promise of work. He made the trip. He found a backpackers' hostel in London, visited the production company and made more calls to employment agencies that specialise in music.

At the radio production company he was offered two weeks' paid work to cover somebody's holiday leave at £200 a week and he took it. That was in the last two weeks of June 1997, after which he was offered a job as Marketing Assistant. He then spent years photocopying, packing, translating, coffee-making and waiting for couriers.

From his experience with the production company, Oliver learnt that the media is full of very ambitious people and if you want to learn you have to learn a lot by yourself and not rely on others. You need initiative.

He learnt how to negotiate to sell programmes to radio stations around Europe. He applied the sales and marketing techniques learnt during his studies. After a few years at the company he was promoted to International Sales Executive but his salary didn't match the swanky title, rising from £10,000 to £18,000 in 4 years.

Oliver stayed with the radio production company even though his first choice was the music industry, because it was a platform from which to reach record companies. He chose a parallel field when he couldn't find the right opportunity in the music industry.

This is a really interesting part of his story: the diligence that went into making his move into the music industry. Between the decision of leaving the production company and arriving at the door of the record company he took six months of planning and laying the groundwork. He spent the time going to loads of concerts and set up meetings with heads of radio-plugging companies. He thought he would move into the plugging business but was advised that his salary wouldn't increase much and that he might be overqualified.

He was advised to write to record companies directly and apply to their marketing departments. He wrote to the heads of the international marketing sections of the major record labels. So, again, he went through the routine of writing letters, meeting lots of artist managers, arranging meetings and going to concerts.

Oliver feels that it is important to go to all kinds of concerts, both ones you like and ones you don't, because you get to network with people from different circles. Even if you are not necessarily interested and it is not to your taste, you must always be aware of increasing your contact list.

Oliver spent the evenings at concerts observing the audiences. He examined what was being played on different types of radio, on MTV and in clubs. He took note of what people were buying and what was in the charts, as compared to what was played in bars, clubs and on the street.

After a few interviews he landed a job with one of the major record companies. He got a call from the director of marketing, who was very interested in meeting him. His experience in the radio production company made him an attractive prospect to have in a marketing department.

This is the beginning of the next journey. The record company made him jump through hoops before offering him a job as a junior product manager. It took three interviews! He had a meeting at the office of his future boss and was then invited for a second meeting with the boss's boss. He knew he had to really impress.

He was asked questions such as what kinds of music he liked. How honest was he in answering this question? It is an obvious question but he wasn't prepared for it so he was vague and named a few acts. He didn't want to be pigeon-holed. He wanted to demonstrate that he had varied tastes and an open mind. He was also asked to name the last five CDs he had bought. This showed that he was an active follower of music and that he spent his hard-earned cash on his interest in music. He also told them which concerts he had been to recently.

In both of the initial interviews Oliver had to go through his career and explain his choices. It's important to build your CV and not look as if you've arrived at this point by chance. If people see you have an ambition and an objective they are more likely to give you the job.

The third meeting involved the head of human resources, and this is where he was put through a series of knowledge and personality tests. These psychometric tests are not common procedure, but you should always be prepared. There are sections in career guides that will cover it.

Most of Oliver's work in marketing was email- and office-based, with travel to meetings and concerts in Europe once or twice a month. He worked hard and put in long hours every day.

It took him years to get work with a record company, but he doesn't regret having worked in the radio industry and he used his knowledge of the international radio scene. When reviewing marketing plans for the artists, he was more critical as regards the radio strategy.

Oliver put in a lot of studying and hard work; he spent a long time in a job that was not his first choice; and he undertook a lot of research on his own budget (travel, concerts, meetings, etc). But he got there in the end because he stayed motivated and focused on his professional objective.

DJ/ARTIST

The profile of a DJ shows that the role doesn't fit neatly into a box. The question is: how far do you want to take it? Do you want to spin CDs in a club? Do you want to create your own club sound and therefore become an artist? Do you want to add on clothing and products and become a brand? We are used to the pop groups, boy bands and girl bands who started small and unknown only to conquer the world, but we're not so used to the idea of DJs who become not just millionaires but complete brands.

Roughing up the turntables; not making a single mistake; setting the place on fire; tearing the roof off . . . Is this the description of your dream job? The box below explores the world of the DJ/radio presenter Dave VJ who can be found on Choice FM.

'To break into DJing you must break onto the scene with something new: a new act, a different mix, a unique selling point. Get to know your venues well. Make demos and send them to gigs. Don't send your best hip hop mix to every club in town if you live in a seaside resort which only caters to twee disco tastes. Think about targeting venues and marketing yourself. Equipment is all-important. Too many DJs can play in the bedroom but can't work a crowd and read an audience.'

Simon, DJ at Momo's in London

DAVE VJ

Dave VJ began his career as part of a Sound System. He had to support himself financially as a DJs' supplier because getting a break in London was proving difficult. He was offered a job in Guernsey as a resident DJ so he took his city mixing skills to the Channel Island to play Top 40 hits five nights a week.

Back in London for the weekends, his first break was to get a job at Kiss FM through Gordon Mac – the guy who set up the breakthrough radio station. They already knew each other from regular nights at the Kisses Club. Gordon Mac applied for a radio licence (granted in 1990) and asked Dave VJ to join the team. At Kiss FM, Dave has worked with Trevor Nelson, Dave Pearce, Chris Philips and Judge Jules.

Dave was in the right place at the right time with the right amount of experience, reputation and contacts. By coincidence, with his remixing skills, he was also offered a record deal. His sponsors have included Vestax, Redbull, FUBU and Timberland.

Is it difficult to make a start as a DJ?
'If you have the drive, keep your eye on the prize. The hardest thing is not to be disheartened; as in when you get cancelled for a gig and opportunities look few and far between. Keep going.'

To make DJing a career as opposed to a hobby, what do I do?
'If you want to get to Paul Oakenfield level you have to work out the *business* of being a DJ. At this level you become a brand, like Jay Z, and you sell the brand. That puts you into a different stratosphere. To get up to that level, the best thing to do is to make records, get hits, and get sponsorship.

'But the introduction of electronic data makes it ten times more difficult to make money as an artist. You might have to find work in another profession to make money to support yourself. Get into the profession by doing voluntary work; that's how it has to be. Work in community or hospital radio.'

What are the first steps to building a brand?
'One: develop a following among your friends. Two: develop a following in your area. Three: develop a following in your borough. Four: develop a fan base in your city. And five: develop a fan base outside of your city.'

What equipment do I need?
'I just bought a Serato which costs £300 to £400 [distributor: Sennheiser]. This allows you to take your entire collection wherever you go. You can scratch and mix files from your computer's hard drive.

'You need an Apple laptop. It has the best reputation in music and anything else may collapse in a club. On a basic Apple you will have to spend £600 but *never ever* go online with it. You will pick up a virus.

'For beginners you can download Virtual DJ which will allow you to DJ economically without having to spend too much money.'

How do I market myself to develop a fan base?
'Take a look at the websites of the Ministry of Sound and The Black Eyed Peas to get an idea of a good website.

'Invest in your website. You'll need to have money for registering the site and paying for the space. It would be a good idea to set up Paypal in order to sell your tracks. The site will be your market stall, your shop in the high street, the store where anyone will come to make purchases, so get help to build it professionally. You can find a professional to build your site in this country or elsewhere – there are no passports and borders to getting your business started.'

So why do I need a record label at all?
'Record companies are like banks; they lend you money in lieu of the sales they expect you will make ... so don't think you're rich as soon as you get the money from them.

'It's best to be signed to a label so you can get a budget for marketing which will lead to bigger things, like external money from sponsorship, or ringtones and other synergies.'

Do you have any advice about making a record?
'You have to be thick-skinned and be aware that not everybody will like your music. You have to be prepared to try again and again if you really want it.

'Find the genre you are most suited to. There's no point trying to be hip hop when you're country and western. Figure out who you want to sell to. How will you get to them? How will you keep your original audience as well as expanding your fan base? Look at Lemar's ability to do this.

'Ultimately, the two things you need for a good record are a good chorus and a good baseline. You can make something out of nothing with these two things.'

What is your top tip for DJ success?
'Practise all the time, no matter how good you are. Never rely on anyone but yourself.'

'It is a hard industry. My Dad said to me to get a real job; but he's as proud as hell of me now.'
Dave VJ, DJ at Choice FM

There were many lovely things about meeting Dave VJ and finding out about his career as a DJ. He's a happy, relaxed man; he loves his work; he loves that he doesn't work in an office; he has a can-do attitude; he loves that he can impress his son by introducing him to some of the biggest names of the moment. (During his time as a radio DJ, Dave has interviewed, to name a few, Sean Paul, Snoop, Dr. Dre, LL Cool J, Tweet, Lemar, Fabulous, Ciara, Wyclef, Busta Rhymes and Common.) What's more, he lives an international life: from gigging at London's Ministry of Sound, to Jolly Beach Hotel in Antigua, as well as various venues in Hong Kong, the US and Africa.

FASCINATING FACT

'The function of a record company (or record label) is to find and sign artists/acts and appropriate material (songs), record them professionally, promote the records (product) and associated artist(s) via the media (television/radio/press/clubs) and release in bulk through retail outlets to the general public, financially benefiting artist and company alike.'
Source: **British Phonographic Industry (BPI)**

From Dave's story, we can see that he worked hard on the *business* side of DJing, and we can conclude two important points. The first is that you must build a fan base and create a profile. There are plenty of websites that make this job easy for you (including MySpace and YouTube), but eventually you will need to invest money in a professional site. Secondly, it is crucial to have a relationship with a record company so that they can invest money, allowing your reputation to grow.

THE BRAND

Some DJs become worldwide names. They release records and even start to put their names to other products such as clothes and drinks. The following box is a list of the most famous and popular DJs (and where they come from) in 2007.

TOP TEN DJS, 2007

1 Tiesto (from France)
2 Paul Van Dyk (from Germany)
3 Armin Van Buuren (from France)
4 ATB (from Germany)
5 Sasha (from the UK)
6 Carl Cox (from the UK)
7 Deep Dish (from the US)
8 Ferry Corsten (from France)
9 Paul Oakenfold (from the UK)
10 John Digweed (from the UK)

Source: www.thedjlist.com

A good example of a brand is hip hop mogul Jay Z. Here are some facts culled from a BBC Radio 1 Xtra programme called *Can't Knock the Hustle* by Alvin Hall.

● From starting unpromisingly on the street, Jay Z amassed an estimated fortune of $320 million in 10 years.

● His debut album in 1996, *Reasonable Doubt*, sold over a million copies.

● The major record labels turned him down for a record deal so he founded his own label, Roc-a-fella Records. He played his music on the street and sold CDs out of the back of his car.

- Jay Z says that people in the music business know the biz so well that they are like scientists. He combined their clinical knowledge of the industry with an outsider's naive, entrepreneurial drive. Jay Z and his partners stayed alert to new business opportunities.

Jay Z took the following steps to build his brand.

- He started a clothing company because he noticed that, at his gigs, the audience was copying the brand that he chose to wear. The Rocawear Clothing line began with two sewing machines. The clothing line made $90 million in the first year.

- He is on the board of directors for the professional basketball team New Jersey Nets.

- He is the first non-athlete to develop a signature line of Reebok sneakers, The S. Carter Collection, which holds the record for the fastest selling Reebok shoe in history.

- He collaborated with Swiss luxury-watch maker Audemars Piguet.

- He owns, with partner Juan Perez, an all-American sports bar and lounge.

- He is President of Def Jam Recordings.

- Hewlett Packard hired him to sell their laptops.

- Budweiser bought into the brand and employed him as Co-Brand Director.

HEARTLESS CREW: A SUCCESSFUL BRAND
Established in 1992, Heartless Crew now represents one of the UK's most dynamic and charismatic street-reared brands of recent years. Fonti, Bushkin and Mighty Moe are the three core members of the team.

'We're a Sound System at heart,' says Bushkin. 'When we came out with Heartless Crew ... we were thinking like a crew on board a ship ... it's a team effort. In clubs, Fonti may be on the decks, Moe on the mic and I'll be selecting the next record or dancing. It's how we work; we're all team players.'

The core crew combines backgrounds from the Middle East and the Caribbean; rhythms of reggae, soul, dance hall and soca; and a heavy influence of jungle and drum and bass. These elements make up their own Heartless style called 'Crisp Biscuit'.

Heartless Crew is always spreading a message of peace, love and unity, and supports initiatives such as 'Love Music Hate Racism' and 'Struggle and Disarm'. They present countless music workshops, most notably as music tutors at the Islington Arts and Media School.

Source: www.myspace.com/heartlesscrew

MANAGER AT A LIVE-MUSIC VENUE

Laure Panerai is Music Director for Momo's, a central London venue. It's a world music club for members only and has the best bands in the world lining up at its door. It's the only club in London dedicated to world music so you would expect the audience to be very particular and the music director to be quite a specialist. There are lessons you can take from Laure's story and apply to any music venue.

LAURE PANERAI, MANAGER AT A LIVE-MUSIC VENUE
Laure didn't take an obvious route into a music career, but it's one that she combined with her passion for music. She was a journalist and editor in Paris for *Nova*, which is the equivalent of *Time Out*. 'Journalism will always stand you in good stead,' she says.

As a teenager she was always following live bands and all her friends were musicians. She watched as they had to do everything themselves: they produced packages of their music and sent them to promoters; they organised their own live shows; they built their own country-wide tours, then European tours; they existed on paltry finances; and they did everything an agent would be expected to do. Laure's education in the workings of a band came before her university education! She understood their point of view. She went on tour with them and lived in their van with them. She saw the funky side of life on the road.

She explains: 'To be in the environment of a musician is important. You must love music. Also, specialisation in a genre is important or how else will you acquire credibility or enough knowledge? Otherwise you will be lost.'

She's right. You already know where your interest lies. You already know the difference between country and western and hip hop music. Laure's main advice is to build up a contact list in the same way a journalist collects contacts . . . greedily.

How can I get started as a venue manager?
'If you have never done this before or you're new to the area or city, find a music magazine or listings magazine and check the "on the road" section. I read *Songlines*, a world music essential.

'For example, there's a flamenco band at Sadler's Wells theatre and I'm interested in this band for Momo's. I would call the magazine for a contact, and they would put me onto the venue. You make the calls. As in journalism, you're on the phone a lot of the time.

'If there's a CD you like, call the distributor or record label and ask for a contact for the band. Get the number for the band's agent. Very often there's a contact printed on the CD. At least there'll be a name of a company so you can find a phone number. Then you need your powers of persuasion!'

What does the job involve?
'This is a job for people who can keep on top of many tasks and many demands. When the band have agreed to perform

at your venue you have to agree a date and a fee. You may have to organise hotel and catering, equipment may need to be rented, and you might need to employ a sound engineer and organise a sound check. You have to be present at the sound check. If the band members have any complaints, you've been their contact and their grievances will come back to you.

'All of this organisation might be perfect, but it means nothing without publicity. Get a biography of the group and a picture, and write a press release. If you don't have a contacts list of press to send your press release out to, then you must make one. Target the journalists in the music press that you've been reading so avidly. Find out who to target in the local press and local radio.'

How can I gain experience for this career?
'Find voluntary work with a music director. That's one possibility. Otherwise, at university you can organise bands with the Student Union. Otherwise, be innovative and find a cafe in your town or village that will let you use it as a venue. You could find work with a touring agency. Have a go.

'Here's what you'll find out: you'll learn all about making calls, you'll learn about being a diplomat and about holding the purse strings very tightly. You'll also learn about how a band operates.

'As you proceed further into the experience of a venue manager you'll come across bands that are organised, professional and have developed into a functioning entity with a label, a publisher, a distribution company, a touring agent and a tour manager. You'll need to learn about all these roles, how it all works, where you fit in and who you need to negotiate with.'

Following Laure's advice, in order to get a band to perform at your venue you must know what you're talking about. The following questions will help you to assess your knowledge.

- Is the band well known?

- Is the band respected in their genre?

- How many CDs have the band produced?

- Is there a new CD?

- Is the band doing a promotion tour?

- Is your venue relevant to the band's audience?

- Will the band get sales or publicity at your venue?

- Why does the band want to perform at your venue?

Finally, you should always listen to CDs. It sounds obvious but needs to be said. This isn't part of the job that can be skipped!

FESTIVAL ORGANISER

If the job of venue manager appealed to you and inspired your organisational genius, consider the open-air music festival!

Summer festivals are part of our summer culture, from rock festivals to carnivals and legendary European open-air weekenders. People panic in the rush to buy Glastonbury tickets every year. In Europe, festivals have the same line-up as here in the UK – but without the obligatory rain and glorious mud!

MUSIC FESTIVAL WEBSITES
www.glastonburyfestivals.co.uk
www.loveparade.de
www.efestivals.co.uk

My favourite festival is the Larmer Tree Festival (www. larmertreefestival.co.uk), where peacocks sit in the trees and add majesty to the scene, as well as their own brand of back-up singing to the stage acts.

The website describes the festival in the following way – you should think about the organisation of all of these promised delights:

- a unique blend of music from more than 70 international, national and regional bands

- over 100 creative workshops for children and adults

- frivolities and obscure spectacles performed by a variety of first-class street-theatre artists

- food and drink from around the world plus three bars

- a free campsite right next to the festival grounds with free hot showers and award-winning toilets.

In the following profile, Julia Safe, who organises the Larmer Tree Festival, tells us about the life of a festival organiser.

JULIA SAFE, FESTIVAL ORGANISER
What kind of lifestyle do you have?
'I would say that my lifestyle is very seasonal: my festival is in July, so we work very hard from November through to August, and then take things a little easier in between. However, the work never stops: once the festival finishes, we immediately begin organising the next year.

'I enjoy the lifestyle: the slow build-up, the pressure of the impending deadline, followed by the relief and a good rest! It is definitely not a nine-to-five job, and every day is different.'

What kind of research is necessary?
'It is important to see as much new music as possible, so it involves quite a lot of travelling to gigs. I live pretty much in the middle of nowhere, so have to travel quite some distance to catch good music. I am also involved with programming the workshops and street theatre for the Larmer Tree Festival so I make an annual pilgrimage to the Edinburgh Festival in August to keep up to date with new performers.

'Also, I try to visit as many other festivals as possible over the summer, both to see new artists and to keep an eye on the competition!'

How do you start in this career?
'I started in a voluntary capacity. In the first year I applied for funding from the local authority and managed to get £250 (it was 1993!). I sold advertising for the programme, and then at the festival I ran the information desk and sold T-shirts.

'All festivals have teams of volunteers who get involved with tasks like stewarding and backstage work, so this would be a good place to start. For the past ten years we have taken a student on placement from the BA(Hons) Arts and Event Management degree course at the Arts Institute in Bournemouth. The student does a 6-week placement as part of their second year, and this gives them an excellent insight into the workings of our festival. Many of them return to work for us at the festival and we have one ex-student currently with us on a 6-month contract.

'We are always very interested in volunteers who have worked at other events or festivals, so spending the summer volunteering at as many events as possible would be a very good start. The more experience you have, the more likely you will be to get an interesting volunteer role. You may have to start off with basic stewarding, but you will hopefully progress to the more interesting stuff.'

How can I gain experience?
'I would highly recommend a course in arts and events administration. They have many live projects, so it's not just about being lectured at. This would give you the experience of planning, gaining sponsorship and funding for an event, and then most importantly seeing it through.

'There is often funding available for new projects, but some kind of proven record is usually required. Carefully targeting a potential sponsor may be successful, but they are probably going to want to see proof that you can deliver.

'I became involved with the Larmer Tree Festival in its third year, and my business partner James Shepard basically funded the first three years. We only began to break even in the fourth year, and then for several more years we both continued to do other jobs as well as organising the festival in order to pay our rent. The growth of our festival has been slow and sure. It is very difficult to make it work financially straight away.'

How long does it take to organise a weekend festival like yours?
'The festival consists of one evening concert and then four full days. It takes nearly all year to organise, there are three full-time and two part-time staff. This may sound like overkill, but there is *so* much detail and it's very important to us that it's as perfect as we can make it. This takes time to get right.'

What jobs do you start with?
'The first jobs are confirming the dates with the owners of the gardens that we hire for the festival, and also negotiating the fee and terms and conditions. The next crucial job is to start researching and booking headline acts. These things happen pretty much as soon as the previous festival has finished.'

Do you need permission from the council and the police?
'Even though the site that we use is private, we have to have a "temporary premises licence" from the local council. We have to do an extensive risk assessment that is submitted with our application for the licence. This is checked by the local authorities, police, ambulance service and fire brigade, and we are in close communication with all of these bodies to ensure that the festival is safe for the audience.'

Is there a career progression from concert organiser to music venue organiser to open-air music organiser?
'Organising an open-air event is very different to organising a venue-based event, especially if, as in the case of the Larmer

Tree Festival, almost the entire infrastructure has to be put in: stages, marquees, power, water and toilets.

'Although important, programming the music is only part of organising a festival. Having a good knowledge of music, programming, marketing, and dealing with musicians will, of course, be very useful skills to have in festival organisation.'

What was your background before this career?
'I had a varied start, working in an antique business and a publishing company, then secretarial temping all around London, followed by an arts foundation course, leading to a degree in Three-Dimensional Design at Middlesex Polytechnic. Unfortunately, I was diagnosed with repetitive strain injury which meant I wasn't able to work for some time after graduating. I moved away from London down to Wiltshire, and began volunteering at Salisbury Arts Centre, working in the box office and front of house. This is where I happened to be introduced to James and became involved with the festival. I worked at Salisbury Arts Centre – they gave me a job eventually! – for several more years before the Larmer Tree Festival was successful enough for it to be my sole income.'

What are the pitfalls?
'There is stress and strain when a major headline act threatens to pull out. It's a big responsibility to have the welfare of 4000 people on your shoulders. The timing of the festival means that we are busiest just when the weather is starting to get good, so sometimes it feels like my summer doesn't start until the end of July. There are also sleepless nights worrying about 101 minor but crucial details.'

What are the best moments?
'Walking around the festival on Saturday afternoon when all of the glitches seem to have been solved, just observing all of these people having a brilliant time because of my last year's worth of work. That is very rewarding!

'Also, when it's all over, the feeling of relief and satisfaction after a successful festival is just bliss. We get hundreds of emails from people telling us what a fantastic time they had, and that it was the highlight of their year. This makes you feel pretty good.'

What do you recommend about your work?
'I love the creativeness of it: booking the bands and other performers; thinking about the decoration of the site; making sure that the 300 or so volunteers know what they are meant to be doing so that they also have a rewarding experience; and choosing fantastic food providers.'

What are the ideal qualities for a work experience person?
'Preferably they will have some experience, however small, but also a positive attitude and determination to become involved – without pestering!'

In summary, Julia recommends that you take the following action if you want to follow a career as a festival organiser:

- get involved with any festival or local event that fires your interest

- consider volunteering at both festivals and venues

- take a look at relevant courses

- offer your services to your local music promoter: you could help by putting up posters, handing out fliers at gigs, taking money at the door and writing press releases

- learn to use design software such as Photoshop so that you can design fliers and posters.

Be aware that there are also literary and arts festivals, and that organising these festivals uses similar skills to organising music festivals. For instance, if you are thinking of taking advantage of a music-packed life at university but plan to follow a publishing career, you could help out at music festivals in your holidays and gain many transferable skills for the thriving literary festival scene.

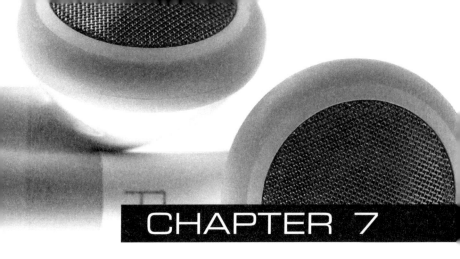

CHAPTER 7

Talent competitions

It's all over the television: *X-Factor*, *Britain's Got Talent*, *Any Dream Will Do* ... don't you wish you could be up there wowing Simon Cowell and winning his respect?

Four Kornerz is a band that has taken part in, and won, many talent competitions. The band is made up of four brothers: Deji (27 years old), TJ (25 years old), Vidal (23 years old) and Daniel (21 years old). Their influences range from funk, r'n'b, soul and jazz, to more traditional Nigerian rhythms from their homeland.

Since 2004, Four Kornerz has shared the stage with a massive selection of artists, including: Joss Stone, Lemar, Ms Dynamite, Omar, Jocelyn Brown, Corinne Bailey Rae, the London Community Gospel Choir and Shola Ama.

To find out about the band's experience of competitions, their manager James Freeman, Company Director for UB1 Music (which is an artist development and management company), offers an overview.

JAMES FREEMAN, UB1 MUSIC
What competitions have Four Kornerz taken part in?
'They have taken part in a number of competitions, both during their management signing to UB1 Music and before. They have won three competitions: Testing 1,2,3 in 2007 (and so they played at the Croydon Summer Festival); ITV's *Battle of the Bands* (and so they played at the 0$_2$ Wireless Festival in 2005); and Heart Beat International Talent Search (founded by Lloyd Wade, who was a finalist in *X Factor* 2004). They also reached the final heats in *GMTV*'s Gospel Challenge in 2003. Finally, they won the Best Group and were Overall Competition Winner on talkGospel.com in 2002.'

Does winning a competition lead to recognition?
'Strategic selection of competitions is a good thing in order to gain access to certain events and public appearances. The Testing 1,2,3 competition run by Croydon Council had record executives present, as well as A&R people and radio representation.'

Might winning a competition lead to television shows, such as *Britain's Got Talent*?
'Indeed! ITV's *Battle of the Bands* exposed Four Kornerz to a prime-time television audience. Not only was their music played, but their website information was also given, which increased online traffic and general brand awareness. As a result of winning, the band performed at the 0$_2$ Wireless Festival in 2005.

'After Testing 1,2,3 in 2007, the local press (including *Croydon Guardian* and *Croydon Advertiser*) have all been extremely supportive by running regular stories about the band. The band was also on the cover of *Wired Magazine* (a local Croydon listings magazine with a 10,000 people circulation), and the magazine ran a full-length interview with them. The local football team, Crystal Palace, invited Four Kornerz to perform at half time during one of their home matches in front of over 20,000 football fans.'

Four Kornerz has played concerts with some megastars. How did they get noticed?
'This is where good management comes in. It is more professional to have someone representing you wherever possible. That agent or manager will be responsible for marketing and promoting your product.

'For example, Four Kornerz featured in the Young Voices tour 2005/06, along with acts like Joss Stone, Lemar and Ms Dynamite, because of a personal recommendation from someone who had seen the band perform at the Jazz Café a few months earlier. From there, I had to pitch the band to the tour promoter with a press kit which included a CD and promotion DVD visuals like flyer and poster materials. A press kit has to include anything you feel would best represent the act and make it stand out. Then followed a couple of phone calls and a meeting and the deal was done!'

Any final words of advice about competitions?
'Never underestimate the power of local support. With independent acts it is about building a solid fan base and where better to start than in your home town? Everyone loves a local hero and to see someone from your area doing positive things and making great progress instils pride into any neighbourhood.

'From there, you look at your regional platforms (the borough), and eventually hit national level. By then you've amassed a strong following to ensure success in the release of any product.

'When taking part in competitions, just remember to believe in yourself and work hard at what you do. The entertainment industry is such that a lot of your success is hinged on someone's personal opinion and you have to develop a sense of focus. You almost need to become thick-skinned and not let criticism get you down.

'Take all feedback on board. Recognise when feedback includes useful comments. For example, if you hear "watch your singing key" a few times, then perhaps doing a series of vocal lessons is a good investment in order to address that area and make you stronger.'

CHAPTER 6

Changes in technology

By now you'll have got the idea that this is an industry of shifting sands and that it is up to you to spend the necessary money on computer hardware and software to take advantage of new opportunities in the music business.

It is up to you to take the opportunities, to promote yourself, to get the training, and to know about the latest developments and the newest technologies. The era of the record company which controlled the music business from band to studio to distribution, and influenced radio stations, gigs and chart exposure, are long gone. If you have an attitude of self-sufficiency, you will be well armed for the constant changes. If you view record labels and radio as the main means of making a living from music, you are years out of date.

'2007 could genuinely be the beginning of a new era. The majors are finally giving up on preventative DRM [Digital Rights Management], while it's becoming increasingly clear that the decline in the recorded music market will only be partially offset by the digital download market.'

www.musictank.co.uk

The 'F word' has made its way into the boardroom: *filesharing*. Most of the children of board members do it. Most of them, I'm sure, do it legally. The suited executives want to license it and help it to grow in a legal manner that makes revenue for them.

According to the quote from MusicTank above, there are falling recorded music sales: the digital download market is the new reality and filesharing has to be embraced by the companies that have the most to lose. The music market itself is not shrinking; more bands with many ways of promoting themselves are coming forward and the scene is more vibrant and varied than it has ever been.

'But filesharing isn't purely about downloading from various P2P and Bittorrent sites – people are bluetoothing tracks, using messenger, email and file-transfer services, sideloading to mobile, sharing whole hard drives – and the list is set to grow.'

www.musictank.co.uk

Edgar Bronfman Jr, Warner's Chairman and Chief Executive, talks about the group being transformed from a traditional record business into a 'music-based content company'.

It is a challenging environment. Every day in the press there will be stories about decreasing profits, rampant piracy, restructuring and job losses. But don't forget that 'downsizing' and 'restructuring' do not mean 'decline'. 'Metamorphosis' is a more appropriate word – like a caterpillar into a butterfly! The spotlight is on those who are young enough to be unconvinced and unfazed by the traditional power of the major companies who have ruled the roost.

As a teenager today, you will have the ability to see the industry in a new light: you will have full appreciation of the computer-dominated world of music and you will be unencumbered by the romantic attachment to buying and owning physical records and CDs. As such, you will have more to offer the industry than someone with a stodgy view of how the industry used to be. A new mindset is necessary to take the industry forward.

Record companies used to be all about records. Then they were all about CDs. They used to control the artist, the rights and the distribution. Now senior executives are talking about the death of the CD and are turning their attention to building a whole new model based on internet music platforms and advertising-supported music and videos on mobile phones.

MusicTank, a business development network based at Westminster University, says that there has to be a rebalancing of the relationship between the business and the fan. Fans should be encouraged to do whatever they want with music and artists have to be paid according to usage.

Other UK industries are looking at the emerging markets of China and India. How is the music industry dealing with these opportunities? What are their tastes? What are the legal frameworks? What are the ways into the new arenas?

'2007 is already looking like a strong contender for Year Zero as far as attitudes towards digital music go. The majors are finally beginning to give up on preventative DRM [Digital Rights Management], giving music fans the convenience and interoperability they have come to expect from MP3s.'

www.musictank.co.uk

A new mindset is needed not just for new job opportunities, but also in the old job opportunities. Just to get to the starting blocks you need:

- familiarity with industry changes

- knowledge of relevant technology

- evidence of interest and involvement

- proof of MySpace-type self-promotion.

However, you should remember that, although new technology is important in the music industry, if you want to specialise in the area of new technology, then you should follow another career path. If this is the case, your degree will be in electrical and computer engineering; your apprenticeship will be with technology firms; and your heroes will be people like World Wide Web inventor Tim Berners-Lee and Napster's inventor Shawn Fanning.

You'll be following the news that companies in media and technology are collaborating and inventing technology to allow listeners to purchase music directly from DAB digital radios, and you'll be maintaining the same interest and enthusiasm as all the people wanting to get into the music industry.

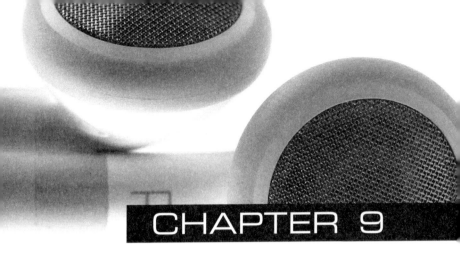

CHAPTER 9

Training and jobs

This chapter describes the kind of qualifications, courses and training you will need to get into the music industry. It then looks at recruitment and typical salaries, with tips on finding a job and writing your CV.

FURTHER EDUCATION

If you decide to go to university or other further education, it's important to spend your spare time productively. It really doesn't matter what you choose to study (Latin, Russian, engineering or politics), as long as you're following a real interest (and not just pleasing your parents!). There are plenty of ways to build up relevant experience while studying that will contribute towards a sparkling CV.

Sam Eldridge (see pages 58–61) comments on his time at university: 'I wrote for student newspapers and for the BBC in the north-east, and I had a student radio show, all of which were instrumental in building up my CV for the music business. Most major record companies also have student reps and this is a great way to become actively involved with a company outside of the usual work experience. Plus I did a lot of work experience: at ad agencies that dealt with Sony, and at Virgin Books where I wrote about the best music stores in London.'

'There are now in excess of 500 different possible courses at over 200 establishments.'

British Recorded Music Industry (BPI), Music Education Directory

University offers the first steps to leaving home, the first experience of independence and the opportunity to find your vocation in life, but given that funding is such a sharp concern, you'll be wondering if a degree is the best route into the biz. You should also remember that there are shorter vocational courses, as well as part-time and evening options. If at all possible, you need to invest in your future.

INFORMATION ABOUT COURSES

The *Music Education Directory*, produced by the BPI (www.bpi-med.co.uk), lists many courses, from evening class tasters to postgraduate qualifications. You can find courses covering all aspects of the industry, including business/sociology, creative/instrumental and tech/audio engineering.

The directory covers degree courses, college courses and training. You'll find information about application details, interview times, audition and enrolment dates and procedures, and entry requirements. The table below shows a sample entry.

Access to Music Tel: 0800 281 842 Fax: 0116 255 1938 Web: accesstomusic.co.uk	Rockschool/Access to Music diplomas for music practitioners Access to Music is a national designer and provider of popular music education in the UK, offering courses from beginner level through to degree. It bridges the gap between education and the music industry by developing relevant skills and promoting music opportunity. Courses include Performing Musician, Creative Music Producer, Vocal Artist, Music Educator, Artist Development Programme and Degree course.	OCN Level 1, 1yrs, 20 st's, Level 2, 1 yrs, 25 st's, Level 3, 2 yrs, 30 st's. Music practice – Apply Jan. Mus. Fac's' lengths/dates vary, enrol Sept. No prev. qual./exp. nec. Interview/audition

Est 1992, Martin Smith, UK

The directory is a wonderful one-stop shop and there is even an advice page to read before you look at the course details. It recommends that you assess each course by considering:

- the interaction of the course with the industry

- the success of past course graduates in getting jobs

- the quality of the training facilities.

The directory is sponsored by the PRS, the MCPS, BMR, PPL, the Musicians' Union, the IRMA and the FMC. Further details about all of these organisations can be found in Chapter 11.

Access To Music (www.access-to-music.co.uk) shows where you can find a course or a music centre near you. It lists all full-time further and higher education courses, as well as part-time courses run at weekends and evenings. Most of the courses are government funded (from the Learning and Skills Council), which makes them free of charge or subsidised. Access To Music also claims that all its courses are custom designed by musicians, for musicians.

Hot Courses (www.hotcourses.com) will help you to find any kind of course anywhere in the country. It claims to provide 'the largest and most accurate course database available'.

INTERVIEWS

Treat your interview for a course in the same way that you would treat an interview for a job. Don't skip on the research. Prove that you are making a considered choice and that you have thought about course content, the reputation of the institution, the track record of the teachers, the employment outcomes of the graduates (the department will hold statistics), and the contacts with the industry and possible placements.

OTHER TRAINING OPPORTUNITIES

Youth Music Action Zones are active in some of Britain's most disadvantaged areas. It's a national charity to help people up to 18 years of age to make music. By 2006, it aimed to have involved more than one million children and young people in its music-making opportunities. The National Lottery and the Arts Council of England are among its sources of funding.

The website (www.youthmusic.org.uk) gives profiles of various jobs in the industry, but there's a lot more than that on offer. Here's a few of the projects:

● Sound Futures in Birmingham stages DJ and sound production lessons

● Remix in Bristol and Gloucester had Courtney Pine conduct workshops

● Gmmaz in Manchester set up a recording studio

● Music4u in the Humber region runs percussion projects

● Sound Connections in London hosts music business seminars

● Mzone in Liverpool runs a drumming programme.

The **Brit School** (www.brit.croydon.sch.uk) is Britain's only free Performing Arts and Technology School. It's a vocational school for 14- to 19-year-olds.

Learn Direct (www.learndirect-advice.co.uk) offers help and advice about finding work and has very comprehensive profiles on individual jobs. The site has, at present, over 700 jobs.

The **BBC Radio 1** 'One Music' website (www.bbc.co.uk/radio1/onemusic) provides information about getting into the music industry. The site covers all areas of music making, from advice about putting on a gig, to listening to unsigned bands and writing a review, as well as listing industry jobs.

WHAT'S THE BEST ROUTE FOR ME?

The profiles in this book represent a wide range of skilled people, from those who have an academic education up to degree level, to those who have acquired their skills through schemes, community centres and evening classes, and including those who are fully self-taught.

- Ahmad Dayes is a music producer; after A levels, he found that the Midi Music Company offered the practical training he needed. Ahmad discovered that MMC was fully equipped with industry-standard equipment, that classes were taught by people still working in the industry, and that contacts offered by the centre ensured ready and supported access to work placements and jobs.

- Sam Eldridge is a band manger; he studied English Literature at degree level and made full use of his free time to pursue his musical interests.

- Neil Gardener is a teacher at the Gateway School of Recording and Music Technology; he says that training is essential to be a sound engineer.

- Moshik is a sound engineer and musician/composer; he decided against formal education.

- Laure Panerai is a music director; she has a master's degree in Contemporary History.

- Julia Safe is a festival organiser; she studied Three-Dimensional Design at degree level, and would recommend a course in arts and event production.

- Alice Schofield works for Anglo Plugging; she doesn't necessarily look for formal qualifications in work experience candidates, but values office skills and a confident manner.

- Andrea Terrano has his own studio; he studied sound engineering, became a teacher and took short courses wherever possible.

- Oliver X is a head buyer for a music distribution company; he studied European Business and Technology at degree level, followed by a master's degree in Sales and Marketing.

These profiles only go to prove that there are no hard rules to follow to get into, and be successful in, the music industry. You must do what is right for you. You will need hard work and commitment, as well as qualifications and training.

NEXT STEPS

If you wanted a job in teaching it is very clear that entry levels would match your qualifications from degree onwards. However, music and media careers are less straightforward and, although further education promises higher pay in the long term, it doesn't promise straightforward entry in the short term.

Graduate schemes are run by major record labels. Warner Music has been mentioned as a company with an extensive graduate scheme programme (see pages 15–16). Handle Recruitment (www.handle.co.uk) has this advice about graduate schemes: 'Every week we receive hundreds of unsolicited applications from graduates and college leavers wanting to work in the music industry. In fact, there are now many universities and colleges running specific music industry courses. To be successful, music must be an important part of your life. You will need to demonstrate that you're *actively involved* in music.'

Active involvement in music may include:

● being a member of a university entertainments committee

● promoting bands or clubs

● being an avid gig-goer

● doing voluntary work experience in a record company

● working in a record shop at weekends.

Work experience through school and volunteer experience in the holidays is an excellent way to prove that music is part of your life. We've looked at many aspects of work experience in Chapter 5, including the ability to conduct yourself impressively in the world of work. Ask a teacher to go through some role plays so that you can practice asking questions, such as how to ask for help or how to put yourself forward when you run out of things to do. It's important to make the most of every opportunity.

Career and work placement advice can be found on the BBC 'One Life' website (www.bbc.co.uk/onelife). Before taking the job, research the roles and read job profiles. These can be found on the BBC Radio 1 'One Music' website (www.bbc.co.uk/radio1/onemusic).

JOB WEBSITES
The following websites are good sources when you are looking for a job:

- The Big Choice (www.thebigchoice.com): student and graduate job site featuring volunteer and entry-level jobs

- Handle Recruitment (www.handle.co.uk): claims 'the most exciting roles in the music, entertainment and media industries since 1978'

- Music Week (www.musicweek.com/jobs): great place to keep up with the latest news in the industry as well as finding work and viewing classified ads

- Sony BMG Music Entertainment (www.sonybmgmusic.co.uk).

SALARIES
Here is a list of music industry jobs that I found on the website of Reed (www.reed.co.uk), to give you an indication of salaries:

- advertisement sales executive: £15,000–£25,000 pa, OTE (over target earnings)

- financial accountant: £40,000–£50,000 pa

- HR administrator for a record label: £20,000–£25,000 pa

- licensing operations researcher: £17,474 pa, inc. benefits

- personal assistant: £10.00–£10.50 per hour

- production assistant: up to £23,000 pa

- receptionist/administrator: £16,000–£18,000 pa.

The box below reproduces a job advert from the same website in greater detail.

EXAMPLE OF A JOB ADVERT
Royalties Manager
Job location: London, south-east England
Salary: £28,000 pa
Job type: Permanent
An established independent label/music publisher is looking for an experienced music publishing royalties manager to join their busy team. Dealing with a broad range of activities from statement production through to payment runs and staff training, this is a great opportunity to join an established team and really add value in a busy music publishing environment.
Source: www.reed.co.uk

YOUR CV

Another book published by Trotman, *Winning CVs for First-time Job Hunters*, by a working careers adviser called Kathleen Houston has examples of CVs, with advice about content, length and the best font to use. There's also a quiz to help you prepare for writing your CV.

According to Kathleen Houston, the basis of a compelling CV is 'your three strongest and best personality qualities; your strongest and best skills, with examples to prove them; and your experience in any work environment or your key transferable skills'. Having established these building blocks, she helps you build the 'template CV' and covering letter.

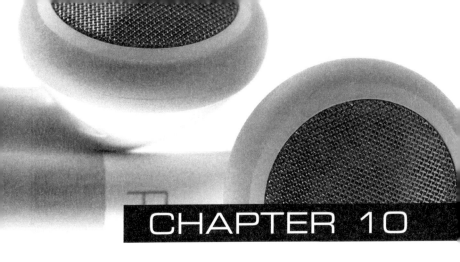

CHAPTER 10

The awards

For those who make it into the industry with passion and single-mindedness, there are award events around every corner. Here are just a few of the best-known ones: World Music Awards, MTV Awards, The Brit Awards and Grammy Awards. There are many more awards, all highly respected, hosted by the music-industry magazines and periodicals.

Which one will you go for?

The Music Week awards honour the best in the business and its categories include: Booking Agent of the Year, Concert Promoter of the Year, Producer of the Year, Public Relations Campaign of the Year, Catalogue Marketing Campaign of the Year, Independent Record Label of the Year and Manager of the Year. Whatever your chosen field, there is an award waiting for you.

DARYL EASLEA, AWARD WINNER
Daryl Easlea is former Deputy Editor of *Record Collector* and writes for *Mojo*, the *Guardian* and other publications. He is currently Head of Catalogue Publicity at Universal Music. He is the writer of a book called *Everybody Dance: Chic and the Politics of Disco*.

In 2005, Daryl Easlea won the first of his awards (with colleague Silvia Montello of Universal Music) for *The Summer of Motown*. It was for the Music Week Best Catalogue Marketing Campaign.

'It's a great cliché to say "be true to yourself and be happy", but life really is too short to be otherwise. To have a thirst for music, and a true passion for it, for me, is very important. If you ever think you're pretending and trying too hard, then you're best suited to something else. Passion is often undervalued by those who shout loud but ultimately achieve nothing. Everything I've read, seen or listened to since 1968 (when I can consciously recall listening to music) informs what I do. My nephew said to me recently, "I get it, Uncle, music is your football".

'To be in a very fortunate position where I work in the catalogue department for Universal, looking after the Motown and Stax repertoire, in some respects, makes my hobby my job. To be a writer and published author about music also makes me never forget how lucky I am. But behind anybody's luck, for any degree of longevity, there has to be a great deal of hard work, too.

'It was a pleasure to win the Music Week award for Best Catalogue Marketing Campaign. Walking on stage at London's swanky Grosvenor House Hotel was *such* a thrill. But awards are often about a whole heap of other things than what you actually did. Every day I equal or exceed my "award-winning feat": it's just that no one is necessarily around to see it. So it really makes it delightful when someone does notice.

'Just think things through. You probably know a great deal more, or at least the same, as those you respect. And do enjoy yourself in the process, we only get to do this once.'

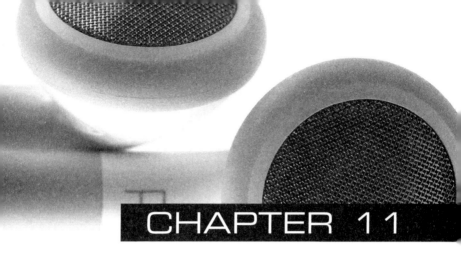

CHAPTER 11

Further information

MUSIC INDUSTRY CONTACTS

Access To Music
18 York Road
Leicester LE1 5TS
Tel: 0800 281 842
Website: www.access-to-music.co.uk

British Music Rights (BMR)
British Music House
26 Berners Street
London W1P 3DB
Tel: 020 7306 4446
Website: www.bmr.org

British Phonographic Industry (BPI)
R25 Savile Row
London W1X 1AA
Tel: 020 7851 4000
Website: www.bpi-med.co.uk
(Produces the *Music Education Directory* and offers careers advice.)

Fat Cat
Website: www.fat-cat.co.uk/diy (Designed to help new artists find out what they need to know about getting their work out into the world.)

Federation of Music Collectives (FMC)
Space 28
North Lotts
Dublin 1
Ireland
Tel: +353 1 878 2244
Website: www.fmc-ireland.com

International Federation of Phonographic Industries (IFPI)
5th Floor
54–62 Regent Street
London W1B 5ER
Tel: 020 7878 7900
Website: www.ifpi.org

Mechanical Copyright Protection Society (MCPS)
Elgar House
41 Streatham High Road
London SW16 1ER
Tel: 020 8769 4400
Website: www.mcps-prs-alliance.co.uk

Musicians' Union
National Office
60–62 Clapham Road
London SW9 0JJ
Tel: 020 7582 5566
Website: www.musiciansunion.org.uk

Music Publishers Association (MPA)
3rd Floor Strandgate
18–20 York Buildings
London WC2N 6JU
Tel: 020 7839 7779
Website: www.mpaonline.org.uk

Music Tank
University of Westminster
5th Floor, Copland Building
115 New Cavendish Street
London W1W 6UW
Tel: 020 7915 5412
Website: www.musictank.co.uk

Performing Rights Society (PRS)
Copyright House
29–33 Berners Street
London W1T 3AB
Tel: 020 7580 5544
Website: www.mcps-prs-alliance.co.uk

Phonographic Performance Limited (PPL)
1 Upper James Street
London W1F 9DE
Tel: 020 7534 1000
Website: www.ppluk.com

Youth Music Action Zones
One America Street
London SE1 0NE
Tel: 020 7902 1060
Website: www.youthmusic.org.uk

USEFUL WEBSITES

www.access-to-music.co.uk
www.bbc.co.uk/onelife
www.bbc.co.uk/radio1/onemusic
www.hotcourses.com
www.learndirect-advice.co.uk
www.musicweek.com
www.sonybmgmusic.co.uk
www.thebigchoice.com
www.warnermusiccareers.com
www.youthmusic.org.uk

FURTHER READING

Paul Charles, *The Complete Guide to Playing Live*, Omnibus, 2004

Daryl Easlea, *Everybody Dance: Chic and the Politics of Disco*, Helter Skelter Publishing, 2004

Kathleen Houston, *Winning CVs for First-time Job Hunters*, Trotman, 2004

Donald Passman, *All You Need to Know About the Music Business*, Penguin Books Ltd, 2004